Martin Faulks has been a student of the oriental arts since he was five years old. He trained in Zen Buddhism in Japan, has a black belt in the Korean martial art, Kuk Sool Won, and is proficient in the mystical disciplines of China, including Tai Chi, Meditation, Qi Gong and the legendary form of Yi Jin Jing.

Philippa Faulks is a writer and researcher of alternative history and religion, with a special interest in ancient Egypt. Philippa originally trained as an aromatherapist and worked extensively within the health-food trade. Her other interests include minimalism and how to live a simple life; you can follow her blog at http://thissimplelifeishere.blogspot.co.uk/

Also by Martin Faulks

Secrets of Rejuvenation
Butterfly Tai Chi
Becoming a Ninja Warrior
Becoming the Lotus: How to Achieve the Full Lotus Posture

Also by Philippa Faulks

The Masonic Magician
A Handbook for the Freemason's Wife
Secrets of Meditation
Henna Magic
Modern Mantras

THE ZEN DIET REVOLUTION

THE MINDFUL PATH TO PERMANENT WEIGHT LOSS

STARVE THE FAT • FEED YOUR HEALTH • TRANSFORM YOUR LIFE

MARTIN AND PHILIPPA FAULKS
WITH DR RICHARD FAULKS

WATKINS PUBLISHING
LONDON

Distributed in the USA and Canada by Sterling Publishing Co., Inc.
387 Park Avenue South, New York, NY 10016-8810

This edition first published in the UK and USA 2013 by
Watkins Publishing Ltd, Sixth Floor,
75 Wells Street, London W1T 3QH

A member of Osprey Group

1 3 5 7 9 10 8 6 4 2

Design and typesetting by Paul Saunders

Printed and bound in China by Imago

ISBN: 978-1-78028-396-8

www.watkinspublishing.co.uk

For information about custom editions, special sales, premium and
corporate purchases, please contact Sterling Special Sales
Department at 800-805-5489 or specialsales@sterlingpub.com

Shihan Michael Pearce at the Bujinkan Honbu Dojo in Japan, who taught me to think about diet and exercise in a new way.

CONTENTS

PREFACE

IF YOU WERE TO SEE ME ON the beach, in the street or in the gym, you wouldn't think I was anyone who thought about food. Nowadays I have very low body fat and carry quite a bit of muscle. People often say things like 'Well, you're lucky; you can eat like a horse and never put on weight'. Little do they know the irony of that statement.

Ever since I can remember, I have had a great passion for life and for food. There are few things I don't like to eat and meal times are a daily pleasure. Now that was fine when I was young but things started to change as I got older. My job included a lot of business meals, and I had developed a terrible habit of eating out as a means of celebration. I exercised every day and I think that made me feel immune to any extra calories. One day, I looked in the mirror and I was fat. I didn't need weighing scales or a body-fat monitor to tell me, it was obvious! I was just like most of the other businessmen I know. I had a giant belly and looked terrible. The only difference was that I had a slightly stockier frame from daily weightlifting. I knew the next step was a heart attack. It was something I had seen in many others. Besides, at 30 years old I should be fit and healthy. What kind of an example was I setting to my daughter and to others in the martial arts community? Something had to change.

As a fitness enthusiast and the son of a well-known food scientist I was the ideal person to skim off the pounds, right? Wrong! As soon as I cut my calories, I started to spend every waking moment thinking about food. It was horrible! I fought through it for a month or two and lost some weight. As soon as I stopped the diet, I went back to my old routine and then the weight went back on, which was so frustrating. I started to realize that the problem was more than just a simple change of habits; it was a complete and permanent change, both in my habits and my attitude towards food.

I needed a permanent solution. I started trying all sorts of standardized diets, including ones where I would eat salad for dinner every night. Some of them had great effects on my body composition, but it was so hard to live a normal life and impossible to keep to in the long term. I kept changing my meal plan, searching for a solution that would work forever, but with little success. Anything I tried ultimately was artificial and forced and couldn't be maintained for any length of time. What I didn't know, and what took me a while to realize, was that my thinking was all wrong. Your diet and your weight/health management is a skill. It's not something that you can cure with a silver bullet; one quick-fix change is not going to be the answer. It is something you need to work at and improve as you go along. Everything takes an ongoing effort: your food choices, your rest and your exercise. It even takes a while for your body to develop the ability to burn fat. That's right, your fat-burning response, if you have never used it before, actually gets better and better. When I realized that, everything changed. I started applying the disciplines and philosophies I had learned from other areas of my life to my diet and body-weight goals, with amazing results.

This book is the result of many years of my studying the art of weight management, diet and exercise. Everything you read in this book is something we have tried and tested and proved to work. The science is sound due to the kind help of my father, world-renowned food scientist Richard Faulks. In your hands you hold the key to total control over your body weight, your looks and your health. You need only turn the key in the lock to open the doorway to the new you.

This approach isn't just for people like me – it is for everyone. Philippa's story is somewhat different. For many years she was really quite 'skinny' and desperate to put on weight. On the following pages she explains her Zen Diet story.

Philippa's Zen Diet story

I was always being asked stupid questions about my weight and food habits, and was continually under suspicion of being anorexic, which wasn't helped by the fact that I had suffered from irritable bowel syndrome (IBS) and incredibly low energy levels since I was a teenager. I certainly tried to eat healthily and was strictly vegetarian for about seven years until I decided I needed more protein than could be obtained from a vegetarian diet. This was due to a basic intolerance of the main protein source of soya, beans and pulses that chronically aggravated my IBS. Many of my vegetarian friends were horrified when I converted back to eating meat and fish, insisting that I could get just as much protein from eating soya and could put on weight adequately with a veggie diet, and so on. However, I then watched what they were eating, and far from getting most of their protein from the 'healthier' options of beans, nuts and soya, they were, in fact, almost always supplementing their protein (and I now know, their calorific requirements) with large quantities of cheese, milk and cream!

So, back on a meat-enriched diet I still didn't put on much weight (although my general mood got better) until I reached the fabled (and dreaded) age of 35. Now, I have a feeling a lot of ladies will know exactly what I experienced – I swear that, overnight from the age of 34 to the morning of my 35th birthday, my bottom expanded and some inner biological deployment of fat occurred. Since then I have had an ever-increasing battle with firmly deposited bulge.

One thing that had been a problem from my teens was my intolerance for exercise – much as I enjoyed my foray into jazz/ballet dance that I did in my youth, and later some Pilates classes, I found it incredibly hard to keep up any exercise for extended periods. I would often feel exhausted quickly and had reoccurring 'flu-like' bouts after exercising for any length of time. I shrugged this off as yet another annoying part of whatever it was that made me so tired all the time; after all, my doctors kept telling me nothing was actually *wrong* with me. Until that is, I saw a different GP and she asked if I had ever been referred to a chronic fatigue clinic. I was not even aware that there was one, but I duly filled in a huge questionnaire, and after six months I saw a consultant who informed me that I have chronic fatigue syndrome (CFS), otherwise known as ME.

This changed a lot, not just because I now had a diagnosis of sorts, but crucially, as of yet, there is no cure for this condition. That really worried me – did I have a lifetime of draining fatigue and all the associated aches, pains and misery still ahead of me? Admittedly, I had already been living with this for the best part of my adult life, and, luckily for me, it had not rendered me completely bed-ridden as it does a lot of people, but it had had a huge negative impact on my life and lifestyle. But now that I knew the nature of the beast, I became determined to try and buck the trend; I was determined to beat it. I did some research and a lot of it was not encouraging; to put it briefly, CFS/ME is believed to be a breakdown at cellular level, causing a whole host of problems, the most obvious being crippling fatigue, and it seriously involves changing the way you live to be able to function better and hopefully make a reasonable, if not full, recovery.

This is where the Zen Diet became a perfect solution for me – small but permanent changes. Because I couldn't exercise the weight off the way others could, without aggravating my CFS, I had to alter the way I ate, drank and moved on a daily basis. With the combination of diet, lifestyle and mental changes, I can now affirm that I have made huge leaps in my energy levels, and the stubborn fat has almost melted away.

We firmly believe that during the writing of this book not only have we both changed our way of life to incorporate the 'small but permanent changes', but we truly think we have stumbled over many ways to help improve the life of those with an incredibly debilitating condition. This book is not specifically aimed at those with CFS/ME, but it has all the ingredients for making changes that could significantly make a difference to those who have the condition. That is, I hope, an added bonus to the amazing way that the Zen Diet approach can be tailored for all kinds of conditions and for all kinds of people.

INTRODUCTION:
THE ZEN DIET PRINCIPLES

What is the Zen Diet?

The Zen Diet is no ordinary diet because it isn't *just* a diet –
it is a way of life. Based on the Japanese principle of *kaizen*,
which means 'improvement' or 'small, permanent change
for the better', it ensures you will never be 'on' another
diet ever again! The problem with all fad diets like the
'Cabbage Soup Diet', 'Atkins', 'Maple Syrup Diet', etc., is
that they don't encourage a permanent change. In fact, they
introduce a change that would be extremely unhealthy to
maintain permanently!

Anyone who has tried one of these approaches will
know that this is not a positive change and that these diets
bring nothing but low blood sugar, bad moods, hunger
cravings, and disruption to life patterns and digestive

function. All the focus is on the initial loss of weight, and then the dieter goes back to their normal eating habits without solving the issues that caused the problems in the first place.

With the Zen Diet it is different: the focus is on the small but permanent changes that you will continue for life. Each change is a positive evolution in behaviour, which brings vitality, harmony and wellbeing. No big dramatic change, just small positive ones. Imagine not being a slave to faddy or 'crash' diets; no more broken resolutions, New Year or otherwise; always being 'bikini-ready' or fit for anything without having to go to extremes. We have designed and lived the Zen Diet; it is not a diet of deprivation or complete denial unless you want it to be, and even those terms can be viewed the wrong way. We need to calibrate our minds so that 'deprivation' or 'denial' become positive things; if we no longer crave what is basically not good for us physically or mentally, then deprivation and denial are no longer an issue – we are not even experiencing them. Social conditioning and status anxiety are conditions that we feel the Zen Diet can alleviate; by following the techniques and advice in the book that work for you, you will be a much more confident and strong person and will no longer even buy into the media hype and scare-mongering that is pumped at us daily. You will just shrug off the 'celebrity' ideals of the 'perfect' body or immediately unattainable lifestyle, and even the bad attitudes to ageing we see in the papers and on TV, and embrace the new you!

What is *kaizen*?

The Zen Diet is the first diet to offer a long-term solution based on *kaizen* and other harmonious spiritual principles from Japan.

The term *kaizen* originated in Japan and began as a philosophy and practice that focused entirely on continuous improvement in the process of manufacturing, engineering, business and management. This became so successful in companies such as Toyota that it eventually caught on and became a sensational buzzword in the international business world.

However, *kaizen* can be applied not only in business but to an individual's everyday life – it merely involves small but permanent changes for the better.

Kai   Zen

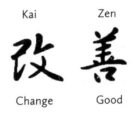

Change   Good

Japanese characters Kai and Zen

But what does the word *kaizen* mean exactly? *Kaizen* is a Japanese term meaning 'small change'. The idea of *kaizen* is to make small but continuous improvements and adjustments, which is extremely powerful, because small changes come without the risks and disadvantages of a radical overhaul of what you're doing. Radical, big changes have great disadvantages. They're risky, they're hard, they're often unsustainable, and they come with a natural resistance from other people involved. Small change doesn't have any fear association, and there's no risk. If something goes wrong, you can simply reverse the change, and with a small change you can't fail. There's no shock value, it's extremely motivating when you start to see the improvements, and it encourages a view of the big picture.

To make small changes, you need to learn about what's going on. *Kaizen* is a philosophy of effortless change, and the tiny changes which are sustainable, and which solve problems, tend to have a great effect, far bigger than the effort put in. But where did *kaizen* come from?

Despite its name, *kaizen* is, in fact, an American invention. In 1940, wartime manufacturers in America were having problems meeting the demand, and the US Government offered a course called 'Training within Industries'. One section of this course was called 'Continuous Improvement', and this small section is the seed of what we now call *kaizen*.

The Americans found that this small and ongoing subtle adjustment policy was the most powerful tool in their arsenal. This was taken on by the Japanese after the war with great passion, and it perfectly suited their cultural temperaments. It also suited the position they were in. They had no resources to spare or spend on big change.

Why does *kaizen* work so efficiently? Small changes don't cause a fear response in the mind. They don't cause a fear response, both in the person forming them or in a group: for example, if we have an aim and we divide it into small steps, we find those steps far easier to do than trying to make one big jump. As it's easy, we can let the change become permanent before we move on to something else.

Kaizen is an easy way to change your behaviour because you just need to make something small – so small that it almost seems silly that it becomes something permanent. *Kaizen* changes don't get in the way of your lifestyle, and they don't cause problems in a big organization. It's about using the power of habit to advantage, rather than trying to use willpower. It makes a small but permanent change.

This book is all about using the *kaizen* approach as a tool to lose weight and to gain health. The *kaizen* diet is about permanently solving the problem. Your small changes add up until you have a new lifestyle, a new diet, a new way of life – and, most importantly, a new weight.

Other diets fail by thinking in the short term. They focus on big changes which are simply unsustainable and often unhealthy. Nobody wants to live on protein alone or eat cabbage soup three times a day for the rest of their life.

The *kaizen* diet is about changes you can keep up forever. It doesn't involve anything unhealthy or unbalanced. And indeed, I don't believe that any diet should involve something unhealthy and unbalanced, even as a temporary measure.

Every dietary adjustment should be healthy. It should be a daily joy to make a change to your diet and make an improvement to your health. Your dietary changes should be something that you can look forward to and something you can relish; but most of all, something that you can feel positive about.

And as you incorporate each change into your life, imagine how much fun it will be to see the improvements to your life, your health and your energy levels. With the *kaizen* diet, you can look at your life as a whole and enjoy all the benefits of a healthy lifestyle. It's about taking the long-term view and enjoying the journey rather than rushing.

No one would choose a big fancy solution that was only temporary. If, when buying a television set, you were offered a giant flat-screen TV that only lasted four days, you wouldn't be interested. So why do people keep choosing diets that are only quick fixes?

Making the changes that count!

For so many people weight-loss goals are chaotic. As soon as they feel they have made some progress, something happens to disrupt the routine, the old habits creep in, and it's back to square one. It can be very disheartening when everything you build keeps getting knocked down. Wouldn't it be great to learn how to make permanent progress? Learn the art of making new habits – permanent positive changes! The Zen Diet will teach you the art of change and the secrets of effortless attitude adjustment.

Starve the fat

How motivating would it be to wake up slimmer every day? The Zen Diet combines ancient spiritual wisdom with the most cutting-edge research into fat loss. It is perhaps the first diet to work in harmony with how your body burns fat, and makes subtle adjustments to how you eat, so that the nutrients feed your body while starving your fat stores. It includes dietary adjustments, supplementation and advice that are clinically proven amongst other things to actually decrease the number of fat cells in your body – all without any calorie counting.

Feed your health

Every change in the Zen Diet is synergistic; the changes work together to bring about a change to your physical health, lifestyle and mental outlook, and bring a positive change to your view of yourself and evolution in your interaction with food. By starving the fat and feeding your health, the changes to your weight and eating patterns will be continual *and* healthy.

Why is the Zen Diet better than other diets?

The difference is that the Zen Diet is not *just* another diet: it is a way of living. The small but permanent changes mean that the 'yo-yo effect' of other diets does not occur – making the changes YOU need means it is tailor-made to your body and your routine in a way that other diets cannot offer. Weight loss will be steady and permanent, and your health will get better and better; it is a perfect way to look after your body at any age and *forever*! By creating positive habits that will stay with you for life, you will not only achieve the body you desire, but also keep yourself in great shape mentally and physically. But we are not just focusing on random changes, we are focusing on the changes that have been proven to bring about the most dramatic change for the least amount of effort.

What does it involve?

This is a book you will want to read again and again. Why? Because each time you read it, you will be inspired to make some more improvements to your diet.

Here's how it works – as you read, choose a *small* improvement to your diet. It has to be such a *small* change that it seems simple and almost silly to make. If it is not so small that it's laughable, you're thinking too big.

For example: you could choose to cut out all caloric drinks. Maybe that's not small enough. Maybe you could choose to cut out one fizzy drink a day. This may seem like an extremely small change, but if you stop downing a can of fizzy drink every day, it would make a significant change to your life. An average can of cola has 140 calories. Now imagine that you drank one of those every day for a year. That's 365 times 140. That's 51,100 calories a year.

That may sound like a huge number, but wait …

If you were to cut out a fizzy drink every day for a year, you would have saved 51,100 calories. Now, there are 3,270 calories in a pound of body fat. That means, you would lose almost 15lbs of body fat just by cutting out one fizzy drink a day. Now that's powerful! That's spectacular! Think of that as a challenge. You cut out one fizzy drink and you hold on to that change until it becomes automatic. By doing so, you could lose 15lbs of body fat; and look at that as a result from that very small change.

What other diet could offer that? Sounds too easy! Doesn't it just?! But it works dramatically and permanently. In fact, using this method you can continue to make miracles in your own body and in your life by making small adjustments. It's just so simple.

To summarize, you choose a change that's so easy that anyone could do it. You repeat it until it becomes a habit, and then you enjoy the results.

In the chapters that follow, I will take you through some of the most powerful changes you can make with ease. But of course, you'll also be able to find your own ones.

So how do I do the Zen Diet?

It's simple – read all the advice and take what is relevant to your life and goals. There are four chapters; each has several parts that give you information and advice on how to deal with all the things you need to do to make *small but permanent changes* to your daily life, which will help you achieve not only a healthy weight loss but a stable weight for life!

If you need a concrete schedule, you can follow the basic weekly plans and use the recipes at the back of the book or even make your own and find which things work for you. Each weekly plan offers ways of changing your dietary and lifestyle habits already discussed in the easy-to-follow sections of each chapter. Not all of the changes will resonate with you, so apply the ones that personally work for you – remember, these are meant to be permanent changes and not for just one week!

There is also space for you to track your progress in a journal at the end of the book – feel free to photocopy the pages to make a bigger journal. You may also like to have a look at some of the suggested schedules of change that I have put in Appendix One at the back. These include an ideal course of suitable adjustments and different courses of change for people with different tastes and life situations, including those who are unable to exercise.

Chapter One

MENTAL CHANGES

ONE ASPECT THAT IS OFTEN completely overlooked with conventional diets is the need to change not only your attitude but also what can amount to a lifetime of bad eating and thinking habits. From the time we are children, we are given ideals and habits connected with food that are handed down to us by those around us. Meals might have been a big thing in your family, either from a positive point of view whereby you had relaxed and happy family meal times, to a more negative experience such as being given irregular or poor meals, or where your parents gave you a hard time over food and your eating patterns. All this can have a detrimental effect on eating habits in later life. If we have a positive attitude to food and our health, then we are more likely to be willing and able to make changes; but if we have been brought up eating whatever we pleased, whenever we wanted, it may reflect in our adult lives.

This chapter includes the key mental changes needed to lose weight, build good habits and develop health in your mind and body. We will also show you powerful mental tactics to improve your relationship with food. With these tools you can create a fit and healthy body; with the power of the mind you can effectively think yourself slim.

Trade in the food kick for a health kick

This, in my opinion, is the most powerful discovery I have ever made in my journey of fat loss. As I mentioned in the Preface, I love food. After a hard day's work I used to love nothing more than a curry or a Chinese takeaway. I lusted after junk food and things strong in flavour and high in calories. If I sat in a restaurant with others, every time I chose the healthy option, I had a terrible feeling of resentment when I was eating salmon salad, while someone had a giant burger and chips. As soon as I lost my belly fat, I used to celebrate by going back to my old habits and putting the weight back on. Basically, I was failing to make any change permanent because I was not enjoying the change. This is very important because it emphasizes the underlying cause of our problems when changing our habits. It's the reward that makes us stick to our change. Indeed, this is not just emotional as our brain is wired to form habits based on reward.

But why didn't the healthy food fulfil me?

I asked my father this very same question and was astounded at the response. He had undertaken studies which showed that obese people when asked to eat low-calorie, high-roughage food rejected them as unpalatable, saying, 'I can't eat rabbit food' or 'I'm not eating that'. He discovered that the enjoyment from high-fat, high-carbohydrate food was as much a chemical effect as it was an emotional one. The pleasure chemicals released in the brain and the 'high' caused by the giant leap in blood sugar had become their food aim. The overweight person had become addicted to food: no longer eating for health but for the fun of eating and the high.

That was exactly the world I was living in. No wonder I was getting increasingly overweight. The only time I felt satisfied was when I had eaten enough to be laying down some blubber round my middle!

Not a nice situation. The trouble was that it was so hard-wired; without it, I didn't really enjoy what I was eating and found it hard to stick to things. I started exercising more, just so I could eat what I saw as a decent meal.

I needed to replace the pleasure I got from the chemical high in my food with something else. I tried imagining my perfect body whenever I ate my healthy alternative, but it didn't help. Then I stumbled over the answer.

I noticed I *did* get a kick when I ate something I knew had proven health benefits. In the morning, when I had a mixture of berries with my oatmeal, I really enjoyed the knowledge that the berries contain anti-ageing antioxidants and that the oats were proven to have a calming and regenerative effect on the nervous system.

At that moment, I knew the path I was about to embark on was irreversible and that it would completely change my food values. I knew that if I was going to move my focus from the pleasure I got from my food to the health value, I was making a simple replacement. I was going to become a health freak rather than a food freak. Since then I have never regretted a single moment. Nowadays, I focus on making sure that every meal I have has an amazingly healthy effect on my body. I get great pleasure making sure that I only put the loveliest healthy food into my body with knowledge of the health benefits and even healing effects of everything I consume. Yes, people can accuse me of being over the top and of being self-focused and smug, but it is far less indulgent than eating 4,000 calories of junk food a day. I also happen to believe it allows you to have a far better effect on the world around you.

Once you make this change, you will be able to see an important switch in your body response. What I didn't know was that it had taken many years of practice for me to train my body to be able to eat such high-calorie and fat-laden food. After a few months of living on a correct diet and enjoying correct food, you will find your body starts to reject anything unhealthy. A few weeks ago I tried to have some fish and chips as a treat, but I found the amount of oil totally overwhelming and felt ill. I just don't think it is natural to eat something like that. Nowhere in nature would a food with this level of calories occur!

So if you only take one change from the first reading of this book, it is this: start to make an effort to enjoy the health benefits of the foods you eat and/or the supplements you take. This habit has so many benefits on so many levels. For example, studies have proven that people who know, or rather *think* they know, the benefits of the food they are eating do indeed demonstrate a placebo effect. So *thinking* about how healthy your food is really helps you to be healthy! But here is the most powerful point of all. One Australian study showed that if people who were eating a meal focused on the idea that they would be losing weight, then their body stored less fat than those who just ate a healthy diet. This principle also works for exercise. So by focusing on the healthy value of food, you really benefit; you also start to get as much enjoyment from the food as you used to from its calorific value. Then you will be able to make the habit stick as your brain learns that it's a good thing to do.

So here is your mission. You want to remember this phrase: 'Make food your medicine and medicine your food.' This viewpoint of Hippocrates really sums up your mission. You want to start to enjoy your meals for the health value, not for the taste or the treat factor. It seems like a hard mission, but you will be surprised how quickly you make the change if you start small. So your first mission is this:

Make sure every day you eat something just for its health value. Make a conscious effort to enjoy it and imagine what good it is doing to your body.

Every time you do this, you are changing the way your mind works. It is about reprogramming your mind with repetition.

How to build new habits

It always seems as if it is easier to build bad habits than good ones, but it is about knowing your goals and making small but permanent changes to achieve them. Throughout the book, I show you how to make good habits and break bad ones using techniques that have been proven to work in the field of psychology.

Habit formation is an interesting subject, and a lot has been achieved in the field of behaviourism to find out why we find it hard to change some habits and others seem easy to drop. Most people have heard of Pavlov's dogs, which were fed whenever a bell rang. After a few months they salivated when the bell rang even if there was no food present.

The 18th-century writer Samuel Johnson (1709–84) dramatically lamented that 'the chains of habit are too weak to be felt until they are too strong to be broken'; of course, it is possible to break bad habits and form new positive ones, but *how hard* is it in reality?

When I was younger, I heard a saying that 'it takes 7 days to make a habit and 21 days to break it', but is this really true? There was a bestselling pop-psychology book written in the 1960s called *Psycho-Cybernetics* by a plastic surgeon called Maxwell Maltz. According to Maltz, amputees he observed took an average of 21 days to adjust to their loss of limb(s), and so he wrongly concluded that it must be the same for all habit formation or big changes to a person's life.

Since then, with various forms of research it has been shown to take anything from 21–245 days to break or form habits, so I think we can conclude that it depends on a huge variety of factors such as the type of habit to be formed or broken and the intensity of the habit already formed. A study by a team at University College London led by Phillippa Lally, a psychologist and expert in habit formation (particularly related to dieting and weight loss), showed that it not only depended on the individual but on the habit they were trying to create, and the range of time to ensure the behaviour became automatic. They also concluded that missing a day made no difference to the formation of the eventual habit; this enduring myth that a day missed means that you either have to start again or that it will be harder to continue, has effectively been debunked.[1]

Another person who really knows about habit change is psychologist Ian Newby-Clark, who emphasizes that although change is difficult (and rightly so in some respects as a habit is often there for a reason, irrespective of good or bad), it is repetition and persistence that really works when attempting to create or break a habit. He writes an inspiring blog on the formation of positive traits and some of the pitfalls that can be experienced on the way at: http://www.psychologytoday.com/blog/creatures-habit

So even if changes in habits can be difficult, they are not in any way impossible, and what we do know is that there are some well-known, tried-and-tested principles that we can apply to make sure that the changes you make in your Zen Diet journey are easy and enjoyable. We're not talking about making huge sweeping changes, as that is a recipe for disaster and motivational meltdown; we mean having just one extra piece of fruit a day – every day – or swapping one frappuccino a week for a green tea; you won't even notice the changes, but they become bigger by themselves. Soon you will be easily having your 5-a-day *and* saving the money spent on your super-chocca-mochaccino to do or buy something much more fun instead (*see* page 64).

What can we do to make those habits easier to make or break? Well, there are a few simple rules:

- **Work on one habit at a time** – this book aims for you to make lots of small but permanent changes, but they are, on the whole, deliberately ones that don't require broad sweeping changes. We don't expect you to do a total makeover in a week, but each weekly plan does require you to make very subtle, simple changes. However, there are a few that require a real change of habit, and those will be the ones you have to do one at a time.

- **Choose your habit** – there is a saying that 'he who chases two hares, catches none'.

- **Repetition** – this is the key to all habit formation – just keep on doing what you are doing and you will soon see results. A habit is effectively something we do again and again, whether it is a good or bad habit – that is the method of formation. People often groan and say that bad habits are harder to break, and they certainly can be because we have often spent years, decades even, building the darn things. Conversely, a new and good habit to replace the old one is merely a product of that same process – so repeat after me, 'Repetition is the mother of all learning!'

- **Persistence** – Calvin Coolidge (1872–1933), the 30th President of the United States, once said that 'persistence and determination alone are omnipotent', and he was right. Only through sticking to something will you succeed; sure, you may have the odd slip-up on the way but if you get up, dust yourself down and carry on, then you will get where you want to go. Don't feel bad about the odd hiccup in your routine; it's not the mistake or lapse that is important, it's how you deal with it. You can either spend days beating yourself up for 'falling off the wagon' or you can shrug and say ok, I didn't do as well yesterday, but today I can do better.

- **Share it** – tell your friends, tell your family – heck, write it in big bold letters on your wall. The process of telling people what it is you are trying to achieve is a potent motivator – they can be your allies, your cheerleaders and support crew, but also be aware that a change in habits can be met with resistance. After all, your friends and family know you very well, a few of them definitely grew up with you! So if you suddenly announce that you are going to lose weight, there are a few who may be somewhat scathing or cynical about your new changes; they will probably mutter that they've seen it all before, etc. If this is the case, use this as a spur to prove them wrong – you can do it, and with support and your own motivation, repetition and persistence, you will be the master (or mistress) of your destiny. What an amazing thing!

- **Stick to a plan** – last but not least, have a plan – which is lucky as you now have the Zen Diet to use as that very plan.

An important word or two
on contentment

I believe that, currently, our society has never been more discontented. Whether we blame the media, our upbring-ing or our general situation, we are, on the whole, a restless society – we are continually 'told' by one form of media or another that we *need* (not just want) more, that we should be rich, famous or have all the latest gadgets and gizmos. How many people do you know that haven't *at least* got a mobile phone? I know some who have not just one phone but several, an iPod, an iPhone, a laptop, a PC and all the various bits and pieces that we feel we need to make all these things work better. They are connected to the Internet in one form or another 24/7 – how many times a day do they check their emails, check up on Facebook, Tweet or just idly surf the web? They don't seem to be able to function without having some form of connection, however vague, to other people. Some people have 5,000 'friends' on social media sites, and, bizarrely enough, they even consider a huge amount of them to actually be their friends! But worse still is that they often have hardly any friends in real life, and the ability to have a face-to-face conversation is almost impossible. We can be who we like on the Internet; we don't have to offer up the usual information or appearance that we would do if we met someone in person. I consider this to be a sad state of affairs. Of course there are some people for whom the Internet is a valuable lifeline: perhaps they are bed-bound or too ill to go out, in which case keeping in touch with people is an important part of their well-being and life. It is also a wonderful tool for allowing us to communicate and 'see' our friends and family who are many miles away.

We could do worse as a society than to cultivate contentment, for this then frees us up to enjoy life to the full.

How does this relate to the Zen Diet and weight loss? Everything is integral – the Zen Diet, as you have seen, is not just a diet relating to food. It is about 'dieting' in other areas of your life; about cultivating new habits that can then be applied to your dietary aims. You cannot expect to get slim and healthy without examining other areas of your life – we are not that two-dimensional. There are going to be other reasons why you eat what you do, other motivations and perceived punishments, and a lot of this stems from general discontentment in one or many areas of your life. As I discuss later, there are myriad reasons for our eating patterns, some of which are deeply ingrained; the process of changing these habits can be incredibly hard and may seem too challenging. But we do have a choice in these matters – it is really that simple – we can choose to change or we can choose to stay the same. The choice is simple, but the actual change can be a real challenge, and that is frequently what puts people off. We often become complacent and think that we are what we are and nothing will change it, but if you look around, there are many people doing miraculous things to change their lives and many doing very simple things, too. Nothing is impossible unless we make it so, but of course we need the courage to make the changes. In the following chapters we hope to inspire you with the courage and belief to be able to change your life for the better, and the good thing is that the changes are small ones and not big sweeping ones. There are only a few people who can completely change overnight and I imagine they would have some serious persuasion such as a threat to their life or something equally terrifying or motivating! So rather than 'eating the elephant' as the phrase goes, we are offering you the chance to have a chunk at a time. When you begin to make those small, permanent changes, you will notice a knock-on effect on all aspects of your life. Once you become content it does not mean you have to stop trying to improve or give up having goals, but the main focus is on retaining that contentment and being realistic and happy about what else you want to achieve; that way, it becomes a bonus.

How to cultivate contentment

Don't confuse being content with being happy, but one will lead to the other. Leo Babauta, creator of the immensely successful 'Zen Habits' blog,[2] sums up the definition of contentment really succinctly:

> Many people see 'contentedness' and 'happiness' as one and the same. In many ways, they are, but it's really a matter of focus. When you're happy, it's really a state of being, influenced by a number of factors, including contentedness. Contentedness, on the other hand, is a matter of being satisfied with what you have. It focuses on what you have and don't have instead of just being a state of being. It influences happiness. However, you can choose to be content, just as you can choose to be happy, and if you choose to be content, you will be happy.

Achieving contentment is a skill as much as everything else; you need to work on various aspects of your life to become content with it.

For example:

- Be grateful – it sounds a bit patronizing, but try to appreciate what you have. Everything is relative, and so we can often feel aggrieved, miserable or feel that our lot in life is unfair, but it does help to count your blessings. You don't have to compare yourself to people who are starving or dying in Third World countries as that can just make you feel guilty for being in an affluent society; just accept and be grateful for the things you do have that essentially make your life better. It could be that you have good health, a lovely home, a great partner, lovely children or a job you really enjoy – you may even have all of them, but have lost sight of these things because something else is taking precedence and making you miserable. Stop and take stock occasionally and you may feel better about a few things.

- When you think you need something, stop and ask yourself if you really *need* it or just *want* it; there is a big difference. Whether it is another new dress, a flash car or just a big slice of cake – ask yourself: do I need this? If you are trying to lose weight, you can come up with all sorts of excuses to have another bit of cake, another glass of wine or to have the fish and chips as opposed to the salad, but if you remind yourself to stop before you indulge and ask whether you need it, you may find that you answer 'no, I don't' and can walk away.

- Find out what you *do* want as opposed to what you *don't* want – try to avoid dwelling on stuff you don't want to do; just don't do it or, if you can't avoid it, at least change your attitude to it.

- Learn to appreciate what is around you – take time out to be quiet and soak up your own company. A lot of people today find it hard to be alone, wanting to be connected to a phone, the Internet or with other people 24/7, but sometimes it is just so therapeutic to be at one with yourself. No noise, no distractions and no one else. It doesn't have to be anything complicated, just something as simple as sitting in a quiet place and letting the world go by. Choose anywhere that gives you a lift, but is relatively peaceful; sit on a bench in the park; people-watch in a café or sit in your favourite chair at home and have a bit of a daydream. Use the time to think about how you want to be, imagining yourself as you would ideally wish to be and revel in it for a few minutes.

- Declutter your environment and your mind by getting rid of things you no longer need. The supposed rule of thumb is if you haven't worn something/used something or even looked at something in 6–12 months, then you can happily dispose of it. The same goes for negative thinking – if you are still harbouring grudges, thoughts or emotions from things that occurred over a year ago, you need to declutter your mind. This is perhaps harder than chucking out an old dress, but by focussing on your present (*see* 'Mindfulness' on page 36), you can hopefully get rid of some of the junk cluttering up your mind.

- Enjoy simple things – having and spending lots of money isn't always something that contributes to contentment. Try to do things that don't involve status or emptying your bank balance, especially eating out. Try cooking for friends at home using your new Zen Diet approach or going for long walks, playing with the kids or taking up running; all are free and, better still, really good for you.

A strange slimming tip that really works!

When you want to lose weight, you need to make sure that your body has all the nutrients that it needs – vitamins, minerals, proteins, roughage and good-quality carbohydrates. But you also need to eat fewer calories than your body requires for maintenance; so it is logical that you take in fewer calories at every meal. I was aiming to do this, and so I started to mentally imagine how much fat I was going to burn from this decrease at every meal I was serving myself. I would think to myself that I was having a chicken breast, some potatoes and broccoli and two ice-cube size lumps of fat off my belly. That way, I would keep the fat I was going to burn as part of the whole equation. I found this to be amazing. It really helped me keep the calories down at each meal; even more powerful than this, I started to use this technique when I wanted to snack. I would simply decide what I wanted to do – eat something more or burn some calories off my belly. It all sounds crazy, but it really works for me. I just focus on the two options and imagine that by deciding not to snack I am, in fact, using up some of my reserves.

Waste, not waist

We all see a value in food. It costs money and it seems wrong to throw it away. If your parents were brought up during the war, they were probably taught to clean their plate. You can fully understand why this philosophy has evolved in time of need, but it is now outmoded and not useful. We are no longer in war-time scarcity, and we are not going to be helping anyone by being overweight and ill.

Likewise, we may feel we should eat everything we cook because some people in the world are starving, so it seems immoral to waste food when we have plenty. However, eating extra food does not stop it from being wasted. It means you are 'waisting' it round your middle – which is not helping anyone. So there you have it – if it's not in a landfill, it's in an unhealthy diabetes-encouraging tyre round your waist; far better to use extra food as compost in the garden.

I found that breaking this psychology helped me make a change to my weight; the times when I had a second serving were where I was going wrong and undoing all the hard work in the gym and other changes to my diet.

Similarly, if you cook extra food, you might feel that you may as well finish it off rather than waste it or store it. This is all part of the trick that we play on ourselves, but the only value of food is what it does for you: if it builds your health, that's value for money.

Remember: never eat food just to use it up – it makes no sense.

Are you an 'emotional eater'? – don't mistake 'mood' for 'food'

We all know the feeling: we have just taken an emotional battering whether at work, school, home, or it's been just 'one of those days'. Bizarrely, often the first thing we do is reach for something comforting to eat or drink, with the immediate thought: 'This will make me feel better!' Women tend to go for something sugary or starchy such as biscuits, chocolate or a big glass of wine, whereas men tend to head off down the pub for a pint or three.

This can be a way that you take in far too many calories without really noticing because your frame of mind is consumed with your emotions and not with what you are consuming. We've all heard the term 'comfort eating', and this is often quite apt because certain foods, especially fatty or sugary ones, give us an instant gratification hit.

Emotional eating is often characterized by some of the following traits:

- Do you tend to eat more when you feel upset or if you are suffering from PMS?

- Do you tend to choose more sugary/starchy foods such as chocolate, cakes, biscuits, white bread or pasta?

- Do you reach for the crisps or chips when you feel tired and can't be bothered to cook?

- Do you eat whilst watching TV in the evening? This is perhaps more 'lazy' eating, but we often mix up relaxing with indulging in empty calories.

- Do you drink more alcohol when you are stressed or upset?

Do you ever open a bottle of wine when you get in from work to help you 'wind down' or relax – what is often now referred to by the media as 'wine o'clock'? Do you kid yourself that it is a reward for the hard day's work, that you'll only have one glass, but before you know it, you end up finishing the whole bottle? The medical profession has now realized that we have a serious problem in the UK especially amongst middle-aged, middle-class women who are effectively self-medicating themselves against their increasingly busy and exhausting lifestyles. Many of these women are those who would never class themselves as big drinkers; they just have a glass (or four) to help them relax after working full time, looking after the children and doing the bulk of the household chores. And that's probably not the full story; they are often running the whole household and helping their husband or partner do their job smoothly as well. This kind of drinker eventually falls into the category of 'functioning alcoholic' – it sounds harsh or even judgemental, but it is merely a statistical fact. The authorities are suggesting that we have at least two alcohol-free days a week and to avoid binge drinking.

From a Zen Diet point of view, aside from the obvious health risks of heavy alcohol consumption, the calorific intake from a bottle of wine a day is pretty high at 500 calories. That may not sound much, but if you have already used up your daily 2,000 calories on breakfast, lunch, dinner, plus snacks, then you are supplementing it quite substantially, especially if you add some nibbles to go with it. We are not trying to sound puritanical; a glass of wine is fine with dinner (alcohol is processed better with food) and of course has some well-documented health benefits. But less is definitely more, and if you feel the need to use alcohol as a relaxation tool, then perhaps you could find a less damaging technique instead. I cover relaxation with meditation later in the chapter, and although it takes some practice, it is ultimately a better long-term way to go – definitely adds no calories and is way better for your health! Use the Zen Diet techniques to help replace not only the habit of drinking to relax, but also to divert you into doing something better with your evenings than draining a bottle. Even if you are tired, just doing something interesting can give you a little boost of energy; take an evening class in something relaxing but stimulating – painting, pottery or photography – or if you want to give yourself a bit more va-va-voom, try a fun dance class such as salsa, zumba or flamenco.

Of course, the Zen Diet principles can help you cut down and replace the wine with something else – have one small glass, but follow it with something soft like sparkling water with a squeeze of lemon, or a lime and soda. If you like white wine, make it a spritzer. Chances are you aren't even appreciating the wine you are drinking; I've seen friends who literally throw it back before refilling the glass. They buy the cheapest Chablis or Rioja and just guzzle to sedate themselves. If you genuinely love wine, get into good-quality ones and drink less; your liver and your waistline will thank you for it.

You really need to be honest with yourself and work out what is causing you to drink. We are under increasing pressure from all sides in modern life, whether it is financial, relationships, body image or the dreaded status anxiety. The media bombards us with images and information about how we ought to be or the kind of lifestyle we should be having. Often it is conflicting and contradictory, and as a society we are suffering from a restless discontent – we are shown endless pictures of supposedly perfect-looking 'celebrities' who earn ridiculous amounts of money for doing practically nothing and the subliminal messages are: 'You want to be like this', 'You need all these things to be happy', and, more depressingly, 'Your way of life is nothing unless you are famous (even for five minutes as YouTube is testament to), drop-dead gorgeous or rich'. It doesn't make us feel too good in the long run, and so we then view our own life as less fulfilling, less glamorous, and the grass looks lush and green over on the other side. Alcohol is not a cure for misery or conflict, and when you begin to make those small, permanent changes, not only will you find that your attitude and self-esteem get better, but you will be less inclined to need other things to help prop you up.

So how do you quit the bad food habit? The best and most simple way is not to buy these kinds of foods – keep your cupboards and fridge free of temptation. Don't be fooled into having a secret stash for emergencies because every day could easily become an emergency. To quell sugar cravings, have some quick but healthy 'snacks' available – you'd be surprised how delicious live natural yogurt mixed with a spoonful of apple puree and sprinkled with cinnamon can be. Or try one of the fabulous smoothies from the Zen Recipe section – a cup of semi-skimmed milk, a banana and a spoonful of organic cocoa is a perfect mix of healing protein, mood-soothing tryptophan (in the milk *and* banana) and a little bit of a lift from the cocoa. But you also need to get to the root of your emotions and try and fix those – what are you trying to cover up? Are you lonely, unhappy with your job/relationship/environment? If you can be honest enough with yourself to pinpoint the reason for your anxiety or stress, then you're nearly there and can channel your energy into changing the things you *can* change, but also make changes to the way you deal with the things you can't.

Here are some of the best foods to help beat the mood binge:

- Anxious? Try foods rich in the B-complex vitamins B1, B2, B3, B6, B12 and magnesium, such as whole grains, nuts, milk, broccoli/green leafy vegetables and turkey breast.

- Can't sleep or fancy a midnight snack? Keep tryptophan-rich turkey breast, plain yogurt, milk, bananas and a few nuts handy.

- Depressed mood? You will need a good mix of B-complex and magnesium-rich foods such as wholegrain cereals, nuts, beans, pork, beef, liver, seeds, fruits, pulses and avocados.

- Having trouble concentrating? Again, the B-complex vitamin-rich foods are highly important, as listed under anxiety and depression. Vitamin B3 (also known as niacin, nicotinic acid and related to nicotanamide) and B1 (thiamine) are your new best friends and can be found in meat, offal, fish, pulses, whole grains and nuts. Both help with mental function and concentration.

- Tired and irritable? It's B vitamins and magnesium again, which can be found in the foods listed above; they really are the essential 'good-mood foods'.

Tuck into a good mix of these foodstuffs along with other healthy ones and you will find that you may well be on the way to managing those emotional eating moments for good.

Mindfulness – making every moment count

You may be familiar with the concept of 'mindfulness' as it has become something of a buzz word over the past few years. It is a mainstay of Buddhist practice, but is equally important in a non-spiritual or religious context. Mindfulness teaches us to live in the moment; it is a way of slowing down our thoughts and bodily processes by concentrating on exactly *what* is happening to us in the present. We often find ourselves a slave to the past and fearful of the future, both things that we only have a limited amount of control over, but which can cause us unnecessary stress and anxiety. Brooding over past hurts and fearful of the 'what ifs' to come can waste not only precious time but, crucially, your mental and physical energy. It is now being recognized that anxiety and repetitive intrusive thoughts can cause severe physical energy depletion.

This makes perfect sense when we understand how much energy we use up just on everyday brain power; our brain needs fuel as much as the rest of our body. If we suffer from debilitating anxiety or worry, then we are literally sucking up energy that should be used for the rest of our body, and this can have the knock-on effect of impairing our health. Conditions such as chronic fatigue syndrome (CFS or ME), autoimmune problems, diabetes, hormonal disturbances, weight gain and chronic pain can all be linked to episodes of prolonged or chronic stress and depressive illness. In turn, depression, anxiety, low self-esteem and lack of mobility can then result from ill health and we are caught in a vicious cycle. Repetitive mental chatter, anxiety or obsessive thoughts can be enormously distressing and tiring. For some people it is a daily battle and one that is not often recognized nor taken seriously by the medical profession. Rumination is a term that is given to those thoughts that continually churn through the brain; they are often illogical and cause intense misery to those who suffer from them.

People with anxiety are often told to 'pull themselves together' or to 'get a grip', but it is a serious psychological condition and needs attention. Often the sufferer has lost the ability to quieten the chatter because the neural pathways in the brain have adapted to the pattern of worry; the mind actually begins to 'warn' the person that there is 'something wrong' because the anxiety has caused not only a mental change but also physiological changes in response to the emotions generated by the worries. So symptoms such as a racing heart, sweating, nausea and the need to go to the toilet are often triggered by the thoughts, which then alert the mind to remember this awful and fearful experience – a catch-22 situation. By learning to live in the present using mindfulness techniques, we can not only begin to calm our chaotic minds, but also learn how to accept ourselves and our conditions and move into the future without fear. Recent studies into mindfulness as a method of helping with anxiety, depression and other mental and neurological disorders are showing very positive results.

By learning to embrace the moment, you will learn which things are important and which can be released. By no means does mindfulness allow you to shirk your responsibilities or evade your fears; instead, it teaches you to be aware of what is real and important, helping release you from your shackles to the past and your fears for the future. Every day lived in a mindful way creates more time for you to experience the 'now' and focus on being inspired for your next moment. If you no longer live in the past, nor try and anticipate what is to come, then you are truly a master of your own destiny, and each day becomes an amazing experience of discovery and inspiration.

How to be mindful

As you have now seen, the Zen Diet is far more than just a diet. A perfect way to complement your dietary changes is to use an ancient technique for calming the mind and making every morsel (whether of food or life) count! Following is an exercise you can try to really experience the concept of mindfulness or living in the moment; this meditation was inspired by one devised by Professor Mark Williams in his superb book *Mindfulness: A practical guide to finding peace in a frantic world*. You can use any item of food to experiment with, especially one with a lot of texture, taste and fragrance. Here, I am using chocolate as the example, not only because it is a favourite of mine, but because it has such a universally deeply satisfying taste, feel and smell:

EXERCISE

Choose your favourite chocolate (dark is best for taste and for your health) and place it unwrapped in front of you.

Look at the packaging, see how it enfolds the chocolate; read the blurb, look at the design as if you are seeing it for the first time.

Slowly unwrap the chocolate, remove the outer wrapper and then take off the foil – what does it feel like, what does it sound like? Register every little rustle and crinkle as you uncover the chocolate.

Lay it before you and really look at the chocolate – the colour, the shape – and then inhale the scent.

Reach out and pick it up; break off a piece, all the time being completely aware of what you are doing, what you are seeing, what you are feeling and what you smell.

You are now going to move the piece of chocolate from in front of you into your mouth. Be aware of your movement, the arm lifting to bring the chocolate to your mouth.

Place the chocolate onto your tongue and leave it there for a few seconds to just melt and taste it. Note every sensation – feel the slow melt of the chocolate, the change of taste from a mere hint to a melting moment of smooth chocolatey-ness! Nice?

Mmm, have you forgotten everything in the world except that chocolate for a few blissful moments? That's mindfulness!

Apply this principle to every waking moment; be aware of the world around you in a way that allows you to be a part of everything, but also enables you to slow down and savour your environment. Just as with all the advice in this book, make mindfulness a small but permanent change. Don't beat yourself up if you can't immediately make every moment count – these things take time and if you suffer from a whirlwind mind, it will take time to calm down. But like everything else, the more you do it, the more it will become a great habit. Start by making your morning cup of tea or coffee a 'mindful moment' – savour every sip, feel the warmth of the cup in your hands and allow yourself a minute or two of pure 'in the moment' calm. Then gradually add a few more mindful moments and particularly one at the end of the day when you need to unwind. You will soon realize that every moment is becoming a mindful one.

When you are mindful, you begin to appreciate the little and big things in life, but only allow yourself to react to those things that are beneficial to you or those you love. Living in the moment is a gift, for then we truly connect with what is happening with our body and mind; we can make the time to deal with anything simply and directly.

Mindful living also has a knock-on effect for your personal and professional life – you will be more focused, more attuned to those around you and more open to new experiences without fear. Your life will feel more in control, you will be more relaxed and able to appreciate what is happening around you without being distracted or trying to do ten things at once. Mindfulness makes little things like enjoying a cup of tea or watching a sunset into a truly satisfying and beautiful experience; in this crazy world, a moment of stillness can be the perfect balm on a frazzled mind.

One example of how mindfulness in meditation form can work towards weight loss was demonstrated by a team led by Dr Carey Morewedge from the Department of Social and Decision Sciences at Carnegie Mellon University. It showed that by doing a short meditation before eating, a reduction in the amount of food eaten was evident. The study wanted to see if people tended to eat less of a food if they imagined the eating process repeatedly before they actually ate the food. In fact, they soon found that the more food a person 'ate' in his imagination, the less food was subsequently consumed. In the study, participants were asked to imagine the process of eating M&Ms, including emptying the sweets into a bowl, picking them up and putting them in their mouth. They were then instructed to eat the actual sweets. Those who imagined eating 30 M&Ms ate considerably fewer real sweets than those who imagined eating only 3. Because the study only used examples of two types of food, eaten one at a time, it is unsure if the process would work to help lower the consumption of a variety of foods in, say, a main meal. But it did appear that it was a matter of habituation and awareness that prompted the person to eat less after visualizing eating a large amount of the food beforehand.

It does show that by being aware of what you are eating

and by using visualization techniques to enhance that awareness, that the mind is a powerful ally in your goal to eat less and more healthily.

Auto-suggestion for Zen Dieting

One particular way of using your mind to aid your change in habits is to use auto-suggestion, a powerful system whereby you use a word or phrase in repetition. Auto-suggestion is totally different from affirmations (which use an ambiguous phrase such as 'I love myself'), as a perfectly chosen word or mantra is used: one that is directly linked to either what you want to achieve or to help shift a deep-seated problem or habit. It could be seen as a form of self-hypnosis because the changes occur on a deep subconscious level; not only is the mind calmed by the repetitive nature of the practice, but you are instructing your unconscious mind to do something directly. This, combined with the repetition, causes a change in your thinking and possibly in your neural pathways.

The word or phrase you choose is repeated anywhere up to 500 times in a sitting, and is often aided by using a string of beads to help count the repetitions. This technique is not new and has been used for thousands of years as mantras or in the form of prayers. The use of beads is also familiar to many: the mala or prayer beads used by Buddhists, Muslims and Hindus and of course the rosary favoured by Roman Catholics.

You will need a set of mala beads or a rosary, or make a string of 54–108 beads of your choice. Choose your mantra to help aid your Zen Diet. Think carefully about what exactly it is you want to achieve.

EXERCISE

Sit in a quiet place where you can comfortably do several 'rounds' of your beads.

Say your mantra in your head or silently while moving your lips.

Each time you say your word or phrase, move your fingers along the beads one by one.

You can do as many rounds as you like, but try to do no less than 100. A set of 500 may take you 20 minutes, but by this time your brain will be taking it firmly onboard and you may well have also elicited what is called the 'relaxation response', which we will discuss shortly. When you become used to doing your beads, you can use them anywhere – on the train, waiting for the bus or during your tea break at work.

How long will it take to notice an effect? After a week or so of doing your beads twice a day, with up to 500 repetitions, you may well begin to notice a change. For some this change comes quicker than for others, but there *will* be change. The more you do it, the better, stronger and longer-lasting the change will be; you may need to keep up your 'reps' for months, but you can be sure that what you are doing is creating a new mental pathway with a positive new change, one that you can keep coming back to if ever you need to top up the habit.

You can do more than one word, phrase or mantra at a time, but it is not as effective.

Bear in mind the fact that the unconscious mind does not acknowledge 'negatives'; for instance, repeating 'I will NOT eat cake' will translate as 'I WILL eat cake!', and you would need to phrase it slightly differently such as 'I will eat healthily every day'.

Examples of words or phrases/mantras to use; you will need to tailor-make your own personal mantra, but a few simple ones are:

CALM – incredibly simple, but when you are totally stressed out, it can be the one word you really need and, said repeatedly, can have a potent effect.

I AM COMPLETELY HEALTHY IN MIND, BODY AND SPIRIT – a really good 'blanket' term and one that is re-assuring and empowering; again, repetition is the key. Saying it once or twice is pointless; you really have to convince your subconscious, and thus your entire being, that it is indeed completely healthy.

MY BODY FAT DECREASES EVERY DAY – this is a succinct and to-the-point suggestion. Obviously, you use it until you have reached your desired weight and then stop, but it can be just the phrase you need to kick-start your weight loss; it is very visual as well – you can almost see that body fat melting away!

Meditation as a tool for change

Moving on from the previous section, we come naturally to the subject of meditation. For centuries, people from all religions and walks of life have used meditation techniques to calm and train the mind. Below are several techniques for calming the mind and also training it to help with your Zen Diet path.

Meditation for weight loss

The practice of meditation focuses on engaging the mind, which develops concentration, clarity, positivity, awareness and emotional balance. Meditation needs practice and discipline and gives you a daily chance to spend time on yourself. Meditation also helps to quiet the mind; many people are able to rest their bodies, but very few people can rest the mind. It is a way of taking responsibility and changing the way we think from inside. This form of mental training is one of the most important things we can do in the modern world in which more of us die from stress-related illness than violence or disease. I honestly see it as the most rewarding and beautiful of disciplines.

Meditation is also an extremely powerful tool in your weight-loss arsenal – more important than diet drink or low-fat spread; more important than any slimming tablet or even a stapled stomach. Why? Because it is the only tool that can change *you*, the person eating the food. Everything starts with your mind. That's the place where you are going to find the solution. Just like a queen leads a beehive or an MD runs a company, your mind is in charge of the whole of your being. You can see the nature of your mind reflected throughout your whole person. How you move, how you think, how you talk and how you eat. They are all reflections of your mental being.

Through meditation you can start to see things as they really are. Many people say they want one thing and do everything in their power to prevent it. Inside them there is something else, some other motivation, something that they are doing that is working better for them than the goal they feel they want. Through meditation you can find a way to see the truth and to find out why you are disciplined in many areas of your life, but not in others. You can meet yourself and make that change, see things as they really are and find out why you are overeating.

But before we go into the methods of meditation, let's start with a bit of science. It is important to start by saying that meditation has been proven to aid in weight loss and weight-gain prevention.

It is not a matter of theory – studies show that along with its significant stress-relief applications, meditation is also being proven to be highly effective as a technique for the prevention of weight gain and obesity and also an aid for weight loss. The first study to show an indication of this important discovery was focused specifically on binge-eating disorder. Dr Jean Kristeller, psychology professor at Indiana State University, and Ruth Quillian-Wolever, PhD, clinic director and clinical health psychologist of the Duke Center for Integrative Medicine, put together a ground-breaking clinical trial using mindfulness meditation.

The study used a very similar Buddhist meditation technique to the one taught in this book, demonstrating that meditation increased awareness and that the participants started to view the eating process in a more genuine way without self-judgement and guilt. The participants reported that they were more aware of what they were eating and felt more in control. They also felt more satisfied when they ate meals and started to enjoy food in a way they had not before. Basically, they started to focus on quality and not quantity.

This brings us to an important point which we will cover in more detail later on. One of the most important factors in eating is awareness. More often than not there is a deep-seated reason for overeating. We have simply developed habits that are not useful and are not really engaging with what we do. Our whole vision of how many calories we eat and how much we eat is out of focus, and we are on autopilot. When this is the main cause, meditation can make an amazing change.

One other study into the weight of adolescents in

America recently demonstrated that meditation could be a more effective weight-control solution than dietary education; evidence has shown that education on diet does not work. To put that into layman's terms, it demonstrated that you are better off meditating twice a day than trying to stick to a diet!

But why does meditation help in weight loss?

Stress reduction

It has been conclusively proven in countless studies that meditation is the most effective solution in existence for stress management. So it is logical to think that meditation would help in weight control due to reduced stress levels.

Improvement of brain chemistry and function

Unlike other slimming strategies like diet and exercise that cause weight loss by focusing on the physical body, meditation may help weight loss by improving brain function and correcting mental imbalances.

Some people believe that when the brain is not functioning correctly, it could cause food cravings. These incorrect signals to the body of course result in overeating and weight gain!

We don't know a specific mental imbalance that causes obesity, but there have been several different independent scientific studies that show how a particular disturbance in the brain chemistry leads to weight gain. Often this can be low serotonin levels (the brain chemical associated with a feeling of wellbeing), or sometimes the hypothalamus may not be functioning optimally.

The important thing to note is that many studies, including one by brain researcher Dr Alarik Arenander (*India Science Journal*, 1999), have demonstrated that during meditation the various areas of the brain tend to work together in a coherent fashion. If you would like to see for yourself, I myself have clearly demonstrated on my YouTube channel (martinjfaulks) how meditation leads to brain-wave coherence.

Most excitingly, some research has even suggested that the increased coherence through meditation becomes a habit in daily life and is present even during day-to-day activity. This means that if you practise meditation, you gain permanently improved brain functioning. This may be one of the main reasons that meditation helps you lose weight. Your brain is no longer giving you confused signals, and your self-control and self-awareness are permanently increased.

Increased food awareness

As mentioned previously, one of the factors that keeps on coming up with meditation training is mindfulness. Meditation helps you learn to be in the moment. Studies show that meditation prevents emotional eating by increasing awareness. By practising being aware in meditation, you create a habit of awareness that carries on into your daily life. This means that you become aware of when, what and why you are eating, and how you are eating, too.

Still confused? Have you ever forgotten you are on a diet? I have and I bet you have, too. You decide you are going to make a change like cutting wheat out of your diet or that you are never going to a pizza restaurant again, and only remember halfway through the pepperoni! Or worse, on the way out afterwards and it feels terrible. But why didn't your brain warn you? Why didn't the alarm bells go off saying, 'Hey, you decided not to eat this or do this anymore?' Lack of awareness is the cause and meditation is the cure!

But worse than the pizza dream experience is the 'Jedi mind trick of hunger'. Have you ever been tucking into a giant meal only to realize that you're not really that hungry? Or that you are not enjoying it that much? Yes, it's another one that most of us have done. Being aware helps you get in tune with your 'hunger cues'. Then you realize you are no longer hungry or already full, so that you stop eating more than necessary.

Studies may show this to be true; however, after 15 years of meditation I am still waiting for the last benefit to manifest in me; if I have a plate of food before me, I am going to finish it! At least I am more aware at the time of loading the plate, so I put less on it.

I am not alone in seeing improvements in my eating behaviour and portion control through meditation. The effectiveness of using meditation as a tool for weight loss is also supported by scientific studies into methods of behaviour modification, which consists of many factors, including social support, self-control, self-awareness, error management, stress control and cognitive behavioural strategies. One in-depth study into behaviour modification showed that meditation is the most effective way to improve self-awareness and stress-reduction aspects of behaviour modification.

Tiredness

We have known for some time that the stress response and the effect of tiredness and fatigue are probable causes of weight gain and obesity – this will be covered in depth in Chapter 3 in the section on rest and recovery. It is not just sleep but also meditation that helps you recover. We have ample evidence to show that when you are lacking sleep, you are going to eat more.

Research has convincingly and conclusively shown that when you don't get enough sleep, your body's hormonal system becomes imbalanced. Most importantly, secretion of growth hormone is significantly reduced, which is bad because human growth-hormone has a large fat-burning effect! The reason for this is that your human growth-hormone secretion is not a constant trickle; it is released in 2 or 3 intervals during the night. It is first secreted during deep sleep at about 2 am and then again at about 4 am. If you lack sleep or have restless sleep, you will be missing out on the beneficial effects of this potent fat-burning hormone.

To make matters worse, if you don't get enough sleep, your cortisol levels are increased which, in turn, also disrupts leptin levels. In layman's terms, if you don't sleep enough, you get stressed and your body loses the ability to regulate your energy levels and your appetite. So how does meditation help with all this? Well, in many ways. First of all, mediation helps you sleep better because you are more calm and relaxed all the time. Secondly, it reduces cortisol levels, thus preventing some of the negative effects of lack of sleep. Finally, there are some studies that meditation may even be able to help with growth-hormone secretion and thereby keeping you young – they are only suggestive, but I suspect we will find in the future that meditation really does help with human growth hormone.

The art of meditation

This section includes basic, easy-to-follow instructions on awareness meditation. It is all based on being in the moment by focusing on the 'here and now'. This form of meditation is useful for those wanting to lose weight because it decreases stress, aids relaxation and increases awareness in daily life. In fact, it teaches all the skills needed to achieve your goals; including impulse control and the ability to keep focused on a goal. Often during meditation practice, you will find yourself distracted by external noises or things in the environment around you. With practice, you will learn how to keep your mind focused, and even use distraction as a means of focusing your mind on your purpose. This is an extremely useful skill in your quest for weight loss when a moment's loss of attention can lead you to eating 1,000 extra calories.

During meditation, a large amount of distraction is internally generated, and sometimes this is the hardest to control as it can be emotional and self-defeating. This, like any skill, gets better with practice, and after a few weeks you will find it far more gentle and easy. You will be able to remain in the moment without internal conflict or distraction destroying your focus. This will be reflected in your outer life as you see the conflicting parts of your personality coming into harmony. This is exactly what you need to help achieve your Zen changes!

And finally, through meditation you learn to see things as they really are. You avoid being deluded and led into different alleyways. Sometimes our minds may try to fool us into thinking a situation is different than it really is; sometimes in meditation we feel we are in one state of mind when, in fact, we are not. It is not uncommon to spend five minutes thinking about tomorrow's shopping while fooling ourselves into believing we are meditating. But before we can train our mind, we need to find a calm, stable position in which our body may remain undisturbed.

I recommended four different meditation postures. Try out each one and see which one made your mind calm and your body feel stable.

How to sit for meditation

Throne posture

This posture is excellent for those who are unable, or prefer not, to sit cross-legged or in a kneeling position. It is the same pose that you will see in depictions of ancient Egyptian pharaohs sitting on a straight-backed chair (throne), feet comfortably placed flat on the floor and hands palm down on the thighs. Allow your shoulders to remain relaxed without slouching and your back firmly supported by the back of the chair, keeping your chin raised and the spine erect.

Burmese posture

This is one of the best meditation postures in existence and one I was completely unaware of before I visited Japan. For years I was using more complicated postures, and after long periods my legs were numb. I also found it annoying that often I had to meditate when travelling or pushed for time and didn't have time to warm up. This posture, very common in Japanese Zen practice, is a simple position to master compared to the traditional lotus posture and will be of use to you for the rest of your life. It also stretches the hips and opens them in preparation for the lotus posture. While sitting on the floor, the legs are bent and the feet placed in front of the pelvis, with one foot in front of the other. The hands rest at the top of the thighs or on the heels. Feel free to adjust the position of the feet until you are comfortable; it is perfectly acceptable to have the feet either straight in front of each other or to let them pass so that one foot is next to the other ankle. You may also have to adjust the angle to allow you to place your calves or knees on the floor.

In the Burmese posture you must pay attention to keeping your legs on the floor. When you cross your legs in full or half lotus, the knees are naturally pushed down. Not so with the Burmese posture. It may take a while for you to sit comfortably in this position. To begin with you may not be able to rest your legs down comfortably, but don't worry about this as you will find that this improves with practice. If you are already practising meditation, I advise you to convert to the Burmese posture.

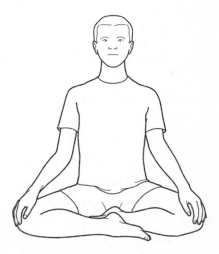

Burmese posture

Half lotus posture

To begin, sit in the Burmese posture. Sit in a relaxed, upright manner. Place the right foot in the crease formed by the left thigh and the upper body. Adjust the left foot forward until it sits comfortably under the right knee. Your right leg should now be in a tight half lotus. Adjust your position so you can sit erect.

If your knee does not rest comfortably on the left foot, then gently press down with your right hand. Hold the stretch for 30 seconds or so and repeat. Never bounce your knee up and down. Repeat with the other leg.

Don't worry if both knees don't rest on the floor or mat. Time will remedy that in due course.

Full lotus posture

This posture should only be attempted when you are used to sitting for longer periods, and it may not be suitable for those with hip or knee problems.

Sit with your legs straight out before you, on a cushion or folded mat to elevate the hips, and allow the knees to sink through hip rotation. Keeping the back upright, bring your right leg into the cradle stretch position and externally rotate the right hip. Keep the right foot flexed, which helps prevent rotation at the knee and ankle joints. Place the right foot on top of the left thigh.

Relax the whole right leg. Now slowly bend the left knee in towards the folded right leg. Cross the left leg in front of

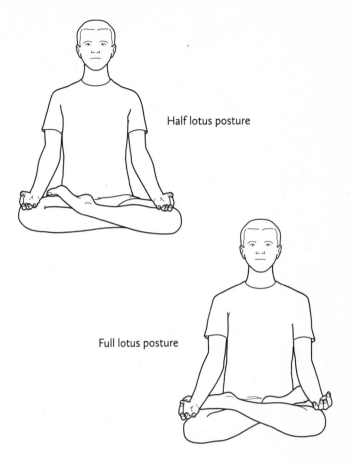

Half lotus posture

Full lotus posture

you. Pick up your left foot and lower shin and gently lift it onto the right thigh. You have now completed the pose. The left knee may be slightly above the floor. Relax; with practice this will even up. Continue to sit in a balanced upright position. The ideal position is not hard to find: just watch your breathing and position yourself where it is most free and easy. Either rest the hands on the knees with the palms facing up or hold them together on your lap. Start by staying in the pose for brief periods, increasing your stay as your hips increase in flexibility.

When your legs grow tired, stretch them straight out before you and gently massage your knees. Cross your legs the other way around and practise on the other side.

How to meditate

The meditation starts with an awareness of the breath. Move your mind to your breath and let your whole body relax with every exhalation.

After observing your breath for a while, with each inhalation start to repeat the word 'Here'. As you exhale, repeat the term 'Now'. Continue with your double mantra. Every time you breathe in, repeat the word 'Here', then let your body exhale as you say 'Now'. There is no need to say either of the words out loud; just 'hear' them in your imagination.

Make these words your focus and avoid getting pulled into other thoughts. You may find at the start that your mind tries to interrupt the process with all sorts of planning, evaluations and distractions. If at any time you have drifted off, don't criticize yourself for thinking or let yourself get frustrated. Just become aware of your distraction and move your mind back to that 'Here' and 'Now'.

Use your breath and the mantra to keep you connected to the present moment. Don't let yourself drift off or snooze. Keep your mind on your breath and the mantra.

This meditation is the first step in understanding how

we can direct our internal experience, and in learning and understanding our unconscious habits. Soon you will notice what things disturb you and what things prevent you from being able to meditate effectively. Each time you notice a pattern, you have found out something about yourself.

As you persist with meditation, you will find a wonderful state of calmness associated with the practice. It is a calm awareness. Don't expect or indeed look for a transcendental state of bliss. This calm feeling is known as the 'relaxation response' and carries with it many valuable health benefits, including stress prevention, regulation of blood pressure and an improved immune system. You may also find that this meditation produces mental clarity and a sense of wellbeing.

It is suggested that you practise for at least 20 minutes daily. If you can't manage 20 minutes straightaway, try aiming for 5. Five minutes may seem like nothing, but make sure you can actually commit to this before you set yourself grander goals – a small amount is better than none at all.

Weight-loss visualization meditation

I believe that using visualization and meditation, weight-loss goals can be achieved with less effort and permanent results. There have been countless studies showing that visualization can aid in the healing process and can increase athletic performance. It follows that it can aid your body in cutting body fat and motivating you to your goal. Your future is dictated by your thoughts. What you think and feel now dictates your future actions. When you use your imagination to consciously practise a new way of thinking, you are literally reprogramming your mind. This is very important because the mental image that you have of yourself dictates many of your actions. When some people try to focus on weight-loss goals when their view of self conflicts with the end result, it brings about sadness and doubt rather than motivation and optimism. This exercise is the cure for that.

In this exercise, you are going to use your mind power to manifest your weight-loss and fitness dreams. As you practise, you should summon every bit of conviction and desire. You should fill yourself with a complete certainty that you are using the power of your mind to reshape your body.

I will provide a visualization meditation technique that exploits this immense power of thought and intention to help you with achieving weight loss and fat reduction. This conviction will greatly enhance the power and penetration of your thoughts to manifest your intentions. While you practise your visualization, it is important to remain positive no matter what. If your mind drifts or you have a negative thought or a doubt, bring it back to your visualization. I have found in my life that when I find it hard to focus or imagine a goal, there are still parts of my being that are unsure about its achievement. When I find I can dare to imagine the whole thing coming true, I know that it is going to happen! So part of this meditation is about getting rid of the doubts and negativity and about practising staying positive. Things are bound to come up, and when they do, let them go and move back to the exercise. In your heart you can feel happy because you are getting rid of such things, but don't dwell on them or let them distract you. It's amazing how the laws of attraction work.

It is also important to enjoy the whole process; obesity and the tendency to overeat could be the product of many years of incorrect meal habits. All this could have come from something inside that needs to change. Irrepressible urges to eat could be driven from emotional hurt or a need for affection. Some people find that when they don't feel loved, their mind drives them to some alternative. An easy alternative is food; from the moment of birth we have associated food with our mother and thus love and affection. Some people ran to their mother when they were upset and were comforted with food. All this started a program in the mind that has conditioned us to see food as being connected with comfort and affection.

Alternatively, the cause could be a genuine love for food that builds as time goes on (my hand goes up here) so much so that one of the most enjoyable parts of your day is planning your meals. Either way, your food focus has become a bit excessive. So it's time to reprogram and give a positive association to new habits and your new goal and to break old programming. To do this, you need to enjoy your meditation.

Practise this exercise once a day and you will be amazed at the subtle changes that happen to your eating, exercise habits and emotional life. Sometimes you don't notice them for a couple of days and you realize that something brilliant has changed or that an improvement has been made.

The Meditation

Sit in your chosen meditation position or lie down. Make yourself comfortable. Close your eyes and relax the whole of your being. Move your mind to your breathing and take a few moments to relax.

EXERCISE

Now that your mind and body are relaxed, it's time for the first stage of the exercise. This is called the energy release. At this stage, you command your body to use your fat cells as its primary energy source.

Imagine a beautiful white light entering your body.

Starting at your feet, imagine that this light brings a cool, relaxing tingle wherever it touches and that, as it does, it commands your body to release the energy stored in your fat cells. Try to do this with a positive sense of command, the way you would draw out money from a bank account. Your fat cells are part of you, so you need to have a good attitude towards them and you want them to listen to you.

Picture this light spreading up through your body, slowly converting your fat cells to sugar in the bloodstream. Imagine as each area is covered that the fat cells are receiving a command that, from this moment onwards, they will be your primary source of energy and that during the day they will be releasing all the energy they contain. This means that your sugar levels are going to be high so that you will not have to eat much at all to feel full on energy.

As the light moves up your legs and over your belly, imagine the fat melting away. Enjoy imagining that and, as the light moves off your chest, see the fat deposits dissolving and how that reshapes these regions.

Feel free to pause on an area that you feel needs some time. You may sense it takes a while for all the cells to absorb the light and all the signals to be made.

As soon as your body is fully covered with light, imagine the whole of your being shining as bright as the sun so you can hardly see your underlying form. Take this moment to imagine strongly everything you want to gain. Think of your urge to lose weight, be healthy and have more energy, and to change your life. Really focus on these goals and then take a deep breath.

Imagine that the light fades away to become invisible; see yourself as you wish to be revealed. Know that this is the real you and that the whole of your being is making this happen; it is just a matter of time before it becomes reality. Like a program in a computer or a law of nature, this will happen no matter what. Imagine yourself being healthy and fit and see your body shape and appearance just as you want it.

Enjoy this moment of success and then let it go. Let your mind move, relax and clear for a few moments. Now it is time for you to take a few moments to come back to the world around you.

When you are ready, slowly open your eyes and take in the world around you. Don't reflect or think anymore about the exercise; just move on to the rest of your day and let it take its effect subconsciously. The ideal is in your mind's eye and will be leading all your thoughts and actions.

Zen meditation expectations

The weight-loss visualization meditation is obviously not going to make you lose weight overnight but it is another powerful weapon in your weight-loss arsenal. It has been proven time and again that visualizing with intent can achieve real results; this is due to the unconscious mind being able to process the information you are giving it and helping to anchor and make it a reality. Jean Kristeller, PhD, a psychology professor at Indiana State University, and Ruth Quillian-Wolever, PhD, clinic director and clinical health psychologist of the Duke Center for Integrative Medicine, pioneered a study in 1999 looking at the effectiveness of mindful meditation in the treatment of those with eating problems and related weight loss. The on-going studies have increasingly shown that mindful awareness and a non-judgemental attitude are a crucial part of encouraging healthy eating habits. Dr Kristeller is co-founder of The Center for Mindful Eating, *see* http://www.tcme.org.

Combining vizualisation with meditation is powerful as it also relaxes the mind and body, allowing any positive mental changes to take root. It is believed that meditation can help the brain become more 'plastic', possibly enabling it to create new neural pathways – in this way we can learn to reprogram our brain to assist us in making positive changes. Just as autosuggestion works on a subconscious level, so too does the message when given visually. It is important to view positively all reinforcing messages that you give yourself; regularly congratulate yourself on your progress and admire yourself for the discipline you are achieving with your meditation and your weight loss.

Rewards

One way to keep motivated is to link each one of your Zen changes to a reward or indeed a step towards a bigger reward. This works really well for some people and is far less powerful for others. The kind of reward that works best is the one that is somehow connected with the goal. For example, you may love the idea of going to the Pyrenees, but have never had the chance to do so. You then can decide that you will make this your reward. However, there is a catch. You are going to go on a walking holiday of your life. You plan all the routes and get everything ready, but you also need to make sure you are fit for it. You may want to go for the walking holiday of a lifetime, but you don't want to run out of puff halfway through it and have to struggle through the whole thing. So you are going to walk every day and slowly build up your stamina. This is an amazing Zen change. You simply walk another couple of hundred feet a day until you are walking two or three miles. It may take you a few months to get there, but your weight will start to drop off and your god will love you. After two months, you will be used to a daily walk, and it will no longer require any effort. By the time you return from your holiday, you will be ready for the next Zen habit goal!

Another wonderful example of making the Zen change motivate the goal is to look at a snack that you eat every day. If, for example, you have a large frothy white-chocolate chilled coffee with whipped cream (750 calories and 21 grams of fat – no, I am not kidding, that's the real figure!) every morning, then you can skip it and have a flask of green tea instead. Then you take the £2.95 that you would have spent on the coffee and put it in the new moped fund or the cruise-to-the-Caribbean jar! After a year, you will have cut out 273,750 calories! You have also burned 9½lbs of body fat! Wow – all this with hardly any effort, just switching a drink. Oh, and you have £1,076.75 in your jar to travel to somewhere warm. That's the power of the Zen Diet – small change, big reward. Just be sure not to drink too much on the beach!

The important thing with the reward for your efforts is that it starts to associate your good actions with rewards. That way, it makes your Zen change more fun and helps make it a new permanent fixture in your life. You don't want to go back to drinking the same calorie-laden belly expander as soon as you get back from your holiday. You want to carry on with the green tea or diet cola and add another change that is just as powerful, like increasing your exercise or cutting out sugar on your porridge. Then you're on the path to your ideal healthy body. So a reward helps by using what psychologists call positive reinforcement. Your subconscious mind remembers the reward and gives you the urges to repeat the action. Then your mind is working for you!

So what can your rewards be? They can be almost anything – gifts, holidays, spa treatments, days off, anything your heart desires … apart from food! That's the one thing you should never do. If you start to promise yourself a cream cake as a reward for slimming, you really are setting yourself up for a fall. After all it's the food-as-reward mentality rather than the food-as-fuel mentality that gets people into weight problems. Remember: the only way you can reward yourself with food is to eat something super healthy. You wouldn't reward your car with rocket fuel instead of petrol. You only put into it what works best. You should treat your body with the same respect.

Detachment – the art of letting go

In this book, we talk about letting go of habits and replacing them with new ones. Detachment is the art of letting go, so it is logical to give some advice on how to let things go. Attachment is one of the laws of nature. We see it all around us.

Gravity is so strong that a rocket needs to build up a speed of 25,000 miles per hour to get into space. To get this kind of speed, it needs to carry a large amount of fuel, which makes the rocket very heavy and that means it needs more fuel to lift off!

Being a human is a bit like this. The more you want to be rid of something, the more you want it; we all want what we can't have! However, we did manage to overcome the rocket problem by making it more light and aerodynamic, and producing a multistage rocket. It had a number of independent boosters that burned out and then detached from the main rocket, leaving it lighter with each burst. You too can overcome the problem of wanting what you don't have by learning detachment. Our mind draws us to strong events, memories, fears, plans. We worry about things that we don't want to happen again, and we fantasize about the things we do want to happen.

How do we get free from our desires? We want to feel emotions, but not let them control us. Time to deploy the detachable-booster-rocket strategy! This is achieved by withdrawing desire for things and letting it fall away. This way, we get to where we want to go, using the energy we once directed at the things we desired.

So we need to learn to let things go. If we view ourselves as being overweight, we have to leave that behind. If we are used to taking the bus, with the lovely warmth and relaxation it brings, we need to say goodbye to that if we want to walk every day. Most of all, we need to start letting go of the foods that are too high in calories or unhealthy. Sometimes, if that's part of our routine or social life, it is hard; also if we really love them. I, for example, love cola, but it's melting my teeth; I know it, people know it, and my dentist knows it. The problem is that it's so much part of my life and personality that I order it on auto. Now and again I reverse my decision to give it up or work out an exception. To be really free, I have to get rid of the whole thing completely. I have to let go of my connection with cola and forget the pleasure it used to give me. It is time to start ordering soda water!

But how do you master detachment? It's a hard thing to describe the process and there is no direct answer. We have to make an effort and find our own way. There are, however, a few hints we can give you that may help.

Repetition is the mother of success

When learning to detach and let go of things you no longer need, be they things that hurt you in the past or habits that you need to get rid of to slim down, you will find it gets easier as you go on. It's the first few changes that are the hardest. You find that if you are not used to letting things go, it is very painful to begin with. It's a bit like getting into cold water: it takes a while for your body to get used to.

Be empowered

When you start to let go of things, you will find a wonderful feeling of joy. It is empowering to see your life changing and you start to find the happiness inside. You start to find the true you and are able to cultivate health. The ability to detach is the best health supplement in the world. You are able to keep yourself free of bad habits that take up your time and sap your vitality. Whenever you find yourself drawn to something you are wishing to detach from, make sure you feel the power of your ability to let go. Enjoy it, feel it and then move on to something else.

Baby tigers

One of the most important skills on the path to self-mastery is learning to stop things when they are small and weak. For example, if your aim is to have a happy marriage, it is not a good habit to lust after other women or watch pornographic films. You may think that this habit in itself will not cause problems, especially if your wife has no objections. But as a natural tendency it will grow. The more you give in to unfaithful thoughts, imaginings and indulgences, the more you will want them. Your urge to be unfaithful will not be realized by these actions, but will rather grow. Remember that you always get more of what you focus on. Having habits like this that indulge a larger urge on a smaller level is like buying a baby tiger or crocodile. It looks really cute and seems like a wonderful idea, but it will grow up in time. Some readers may find this idea amusing, but many people in London have indeed bought such animals and been surprised when the animal gets so large that it tries to eat them. The sewers of London are rumoured to be full of crocodiles that are dumped as a result of this kind of stupidity.

We all laugh at such folly, but the truth is that we all often make this kind of silly mistake with our own life and habits. We can all see the kind of habits that lead to worse and larger sins. The most important point to remember is if you partly fulfil a strong urge or desire with a seemingly harmless habit, be very sure this is not a baby tiger that is going to grow up and eat you. Catch things when they are very small and you don't have a struggle. The best time to weaken an oak tree is when it's an acorn. If you are trying to give up overeating on weekends out, you have to say 'no' to going to that Chinese restaurant. That is the point when you need to resist. If you try to go and eat healthily, you have a major battle on your hands. Likewise, control your meals at the point of purchase, not the point of cooking. If you have ever tried to eat one square of chocolate or a couple of peanuts, then you know the value of cutting things off at the root. Don't open the packet!

Be like the lotus flower

In spiritual traditions across the world, the art of detachment is symbolized by the lotus flower. The universal symbolism is based on the fact that the lotus flower grows up from the mud into an object of great beauty. The lotus flower starts its life as a bulb at the bottom of a pond in the muck and dirt, then it slowly but continually moves towards the light as it approaches the water's surface. Once it comes to the surface of the water, the lotus blooms into a beautiful flower. Indeed, in a way, as all living things come from the earth, the lotus flower could represent life in general. In spiritual paths, where the aim is to grow and change into something more beautiful and noble, this symbol represents the struggle for self-transformation perfectly.

The lotus seed already has within itself perfectly formed embryos containing everything it needs to grow, flourish and transform. In fact, it is said that, if opened, the seed even contains leaves and what appear to be whole miniature plants and flowers. This symbolizes the fact that the key to our own enlightenment lies hidden inside ourselves and that nothing external is needed. On a cosmic scale, this also points to the creation of the universe and the eternal great solar cycle that maintains the whole of life on earth. It also points to the ideal or spiritual world hidden within the material and the ability to access the former through the latter. Moreover, because it has buds, blossoms and seed pods simultaneously on the same plant, it also symbolizes the past, present and future together as one.

However, the most important and powerful meaning behind the lotus, stems from the plant's mysterious ability to remain pure and unsullied. The petals reject any mud or water splashed on them and remain bright and pure. This quality of being able to remain pure when surrounded by swamp is just what the great spiritual masters of old felt was needed in an individual. If we could cultivate the ability to be unaffected by the negative things around us, then, like the lotus with its lovely scent and beautiful appearance, we could have a positive effect on the world around us.

The lotus teaches us that, in order to create something

beautiful, we need to be able to remain pure and unsullied. We need to learn to let things flow over us. Whenever you need to let something pass by, remember the lotus flower and picture the amazingly beautiful future you are going to create; let the mud flow over you.

Remind yourself of your aim

One of the great keys to detachment is to keep your mind on your aim. Many people suffer from aim confusion, and this destroys their chances of reaching their goals. Some people join a company because they want a stepping stone to another role, only to become competitive in their job and spend the rest of their life trying to get the most senior role. Some men work themselves to death trying to make lots of money and destroy their marriages in the process.

With food, people get caught up in seeking pleasure, not feeding the body with the best fuel. If you find your aim wandering, let go of the other goal and focus on what you are trying to do here. When you choose your food, you want to feed your body with all it needs, but with fewer calories so that it burns fat. Any other motive needs to be dropped. I find this really helps with all goals.

Other benefits of detachment

For most people, work is most of their life. It is something that takes up a huge amount of their energy and focus. When they get home, it is hard for them to leave work *at* work and it's like a thorn in their side during spare time. Even when they lie in bed, they find it hard to stop thinking about deadlines and responsibilities. They need to learn to let go. Detachment gives us the capacity to be in the moment, to rid ourselves of worries about reports that haven't been finished and emails that need response. That's a very powerful stress-busting skill. A less stressed person is a better worker and a slimmer body!

Chapter Two

DIETARY CHANGES

Food routine – and how to take advantage of it

Humans are creatures of habit. We naturally develop routines for everything we do – even if we don't know it! Many diets take advantage of this by simply attempting to replace our existing food routine with another, normally one that is drastic and unsustainable. In the Zen Diet, we recommend that you work with the natural routine that you have already created and start to improve it. It's time for a meal-time evolution, not a revolution.

Take a few moments to look at your existing routine. If you get a piece of paper and write down meals you tend to cook regularly, you may be surprised to find there are only about 10 or so that you prepare on rotation. Perhaps a few more that you cook very rarely, but the main focus is on finding the ones you cook or eat almost every week. Include eating out and takeaways.

Looking at your food routine is a powerful diet tool. Just being aware of it will encourage you to cut out that very high-calorie meal. If you have Chinese takeaway more often than you think, that may be the first thing to go.

Now imagine how much of a difference to your weight it would make if you were to replace a high-calorie meal with a nice low-calorie one. It may not sound like much, but consider the long-term effect of this replacement *every week*. You could cut 1,000 calories a week just with that one small change.

In Appendix Two, you will find a selection of amazing recipes that I have used myself. These are formulas I have used to improve my diet and cut away my body fat. They are all high in protein and bulk, but low in calories. That way, you feel nicely full and the meal lasts for a long time so you don't feel hungry, but you cut your calories by eating these meals rather than most conventional dishes.

While working through this chapter, the Zen change to your diet is simply to try a different meal from the 'Recipe' section each week. If you find one you like, it will naturally become part of your routine. You will notice that all recipes are quick, easy to prepare and can be varied. So if you do choose to go down the standardized diet route and only eat recipes from this book, it's easy for you to vary your diet and keep it fresh and interesting!

Changing your food habits

We only have to look at the TV, magazines and any adverts that are flashed at us on the Internet, at bus shelters and on the subway around New Year to know that the one BIG resolution that tops all the lists is to lose weight/get healthy. But often that means yet another weird diet, yet another celebrity-endorsed product or buying exercise equipment that we don't ever use properly. So how do we change our food habits so that we permanently keep the new habits? The answer once again is *kaizen* – the art of small, simple yet permanent changes.

Think fresh, eat fresh

Thinking about food in a different way is one of the first steps in changing your food habits. What does food mean to you? Is it just 'fuel'? Is it a source of pleasure? Does it cause you anxiety? We can adapt any of these things to become good food habits – food should be simple, fresh and vital, and importantly nourishing to the body and soul. Don't think that the term 'simple' means bland or boring, think of it as food that is –

- **Unadulterated** – i.e. not packed full of salt, sugar, sweeteners, chemicals, additives, etc. You don't need this stuff as it alters the natural state of food. You can easily add seasoning and spices yourself when cooking.

- **Fresh** – meaning not having been stored in a warehouse for months on end; buy your fruit and vegetables locally and every few days – food is meant to wilt and rot unless it has been tampered with. Frozen fruit and vegetables are actually pretty good as they usually have been harvested and frozen quickly which retains a lot of the goodness.

- **Unprocessed** – without having been stripped of its natural goodness, i.e. white bread/pasta/rice. We're not saying *never* eat white bread/pasta/rice again, but, on the whole, it is a good choice to fill up on whole grain, not only because it gives you stacks of vitamins and minerals that would be stripped away, but it also gives you a great source of fibre, which makes you feel fuller for longer and keeps you regular! Also avoid 'ready meals' – they are full of salt and fat because they need to give you a quick option with the most flavour.

- **Read the labels** – according to researchers at the Fred Hutchinson Cancer Research Center in Seattle, people who read the nutritional labels on food packaging eat around 5 per cent less fat than those who don't. Just because it says 'low fat' doesn't mean it isn't loaded with salt, sugar or other nasties – many ready meals scream 'less than 5 per cent fat', but you need to check what else is in there.

Get back in the kitchen!

In our modern age we are obsessed with quick fixes – we have gadgets to do things quicker for us, we have meals that are ready in minutes, but haven't we lost something along with the super-fast lifestyle? What happened to sitting down at the table to eat? How many people do you know who just chuck a ready meal in the microwave and then schlep to the sofa to almost inhale it in front of the TV? In fact, we all do it sometimes, but it has become a sad fact that more people now eat in front of the glowing screen of their giant plasma TV or their computer than sit down with their loved ones to slowly wind down from the day and absorb some good, wholesome food.

One of the first things we suggest that you try and cultivate is to get into the habit of making food interesting again: not only the meals you make but also the process of eating it. If you are doing something else whilst eating, you are not really enjoying it, so begin by laying the table in the evening and making your meal a pleasant experience. If you have a family, encourage everyone to use the time to chat about what has happened to them during the day, make it a relaxed and fun time, discuss the food you are eating and savour every bite. If you live alone, still make the effort to sit at the table and enjoy your food. I recall reading about a well-known actress who lives alone, and she said that she always makes a point of laying the table with lovely china and cutlery and having a small glass of wine with her supper. She couldn't see why she should treat herself any differently than if she were preparing a lovely meal for friends. It gave her a sense of wellbeing and was a nightly ritual.

Another problem we now have with our relationship to food is that often people don't want to go to the effort of preparing a proper meal. When I was a child, my mother made all our food from scratch; something almost unheard of nowadays. She shopped every few days at the local grocers, greengrocers and butchers; our milk came from the dairy down the road, and bread was delivered in a van from a local bakery, or as a treat on a Sunday, my father would take us to a bakery where they still had a fire oven in the wall. The smell was indescribably delicious, and after waiting for what seemed like an eternity, we would be handed a piping-hot loaf wrapped firmly in greased paper to take home, where we would fight over who got the lovely crunchy crust. This wasn't back in the Dark Ages, it was the 1970s, when microwaves were things scientists talked about and the closest things to a ready meal were fish fingers! As children we were treated to food that tasted good, fresh and was always an enjoyable experience; it certainly wasn't cordon bleu, but it was traditional whole-some fare.

It may seem a chore to have to come in at the end of the day and prepare a meal, but with a bit of forethought and planning you can make some amazing meals in just 30 minutes. There is no penalty for using the odd can of ingredients or a pasta sauce, but you will find that after a while you don't really like processed food and are happier to make your own spaghetti sauce. If you are a working mum, one of the best things to do is to make a 'Weekly Meal Plan' and have everything you need on your shopping list and in your fridge. You don't have to be Mary Poppins and produce a three-course meal from scratch every night, but with planning you can whip up something fresh and wholesome really quickly.

Try some of the recipes from Appendix Two at the end of the book, such as –

- Salmon and noodles with mixed vegetables

- Pasta and chicken with rocket salad

- Pitta pockets with spicy chicken, mixed peppers and beans

- Hobo packets

- Spaghetti and sauce with Parmesan cheese

I tried cutting down on processed and fatty/sugary foods, and after a while, when I did have some, they seemed really artificial and tasted overly greasy or sweet. I haven't become the kind of health-food freak who shuns everything that isn't totally unprocessed, but I guess I wanted us to go back to my childhood in a way, when it all seemed so SIMPLE, and I think that simplicity is crucial for your Zen Diet.

Zen your kitchen

One of the things you need to do when simplifying your diet and food habits is to have a good clear-out in your kitchen. You will need to get rid of all the foodstuffs that tempt you and replace them with wholesome goodies. You don't have to bin them; you can ask friends and neighbours to 'help' you by giving them any cakes, biscuits or overly processed foods. It may sound harsh, but if you haven't got the tempting stuff in the house, then you can't eat it. I know we often try and kid ourselves that we are keeping some cake or whatever for 'emergencies', but what's the emergency? If you are trying to lose weight and keep it off, cake is *not* going to make you feel better in the long run; ok, it temporarily makes your blood sugar spike or tantalizes your fat receptors which gives you that initial 'mmm' feeling, but you'll soon crash and regret having eaten 200+ calories in one go. It's also easy to think that 'other people eat cake and biscuits, so why shouldn't I?', but they might not care about their weight or what they are eating, and so that is irrelevant. Food manufacturers rely on us feeling drawn to fatty, sugary foods; it has been scientifically proven that both sugar and fat give us a buzz, so no wonder we want more!

In several studies, sugar has been shown to be as bad as fat for causing similar health problems. The University of Melbourne found that mice showed signs of impaired heart function after just 12 weeks of a sugar-rich diet, and another study gave indications that a sugar-laden diet does have a link to the development of diabetes. But the biggest revelation to hit the news is that, according to scientists from California University, sugar is tantamount to a poison and compares with the destructive health consequences of alcohol and tobacco. This is not a new suggestion: there have been several books published over the years highlighting the health problems associated with sugar, including

Sugar Nation: The Hidden Truth Behind America's Deadliest Habit and the Simple Way to Beat It by Jeff O'Connell and *Pure, White and Deadly* by John S Yudkin. The California University study implies that a regular or high consumption of sugar can lead to a whole host of health problems ranging from hormonal imbalance, heart disease, cancer and, obviously, obesity. Princeton University in turn have also done some studies indicating that sugar, when metabolized, creates a similar effect on the brain as heroin and therefore is verging on being addictive. It certainly makes sense to wean ourselves off sugar or at least cut right down.

The problem we have in our modern diet is that sugar is often hidden in a wide variety of foods. Ironically, savoury foods feature highly on this list. The best way to deal with this is to avoid processed foods as much as possible and to replace sweet, sugary foods with something similar, such as fruit.

The idea of treating ourselves has become an everyday norm and is something that we really don't need, but we will cover this later. You don't need to get too puritanical – I keep some very dark chocolate, lots of fruit (even canned fruit in juice is fine) and honey around the place for those 'I need something sweet!' moments. But with all these foods it is quite hard to eat a lot of them as they are concentrated tastes. You will find that, as you cut down on the processed stuff, you will begin to appreciate subtle tastes and not really miss the sticky, sugary, fatty foods – in fact, they can almost be slightly nauseating when you haven't had them for a while.

So, once you have cleared out the shop-bought cakes, biscuits, syrups, jams and other highly processed food, it is time to replace them with the good stuff!

Food cupboard staples

Noodles – you can get all sorts of amazing ones from supermarkets and specialist Asian suppliers: soba, buckwheat, wholegrain, rice, etc.

Rice – try wholegrain (basmati or long grain), wild rice (a type of grass, mixes well with white or brown rice), sushi rice. White basmati rice is fine to use on occasions as it has a low glycaemic index – i.e. it digests slower than processed or sugary foods

Pasta – this can be wholegrain, spinach or tomato (tricolour) or made from ingredients other than wheat, such as buckwheat (a grain), rice flour or other grains.

Beans and pulses – there is a huge range of beans and pulses that you can use to ring the changes in your meals: lentils (orange, brown, green and Puy), pinto beans, chick-peas, butter beans, kidney beans, etc. I know canned produce could verge on 'processed', but if you buy the beans canned in water and preferably without added sugar and salt, then they are a really handy standby for quick meals. Remember we aren't trying to be totally puritan here, just changing the way you eat for the better.

Cereals – go for porridge oats, sugar-free muesli or low-fat flakes; health-food shops have a huge variety of sugar-free, wheat-free and different types of cereals. Use your imagination and add dried fruit or fresh/frozen berries to your cereal. Put cinnamon in your porridge, yogurt on your muesli – all great additions to your Zen Diet.

Flours – making your own bread or pastry is pretty simple, and if you are the one adding the ingredients, you can make sure it is as wholesome and nutritious as possible. There are also some great wheat-free flours available if you are on a gluten-free or wheat-free diet, and leading supermarkets supply some amazing bread mixes that are so much better than the ready-made stuff as a lot of the 'nasties' have been left out. You can even make some really good cakes/biscuits with wholesome ingredients (see, I am not totally anti-cake and biscuit!), and there are some recipes in the back of the book that are great for treats.

Condiments – flavours are paramount in keeping you interested in your food. There are many subtle tastes that we miss when we eat ready meals or highly processed foods as they are often drowned in salt or sugar and we can't seem to get beyond that to find the taste of the food itself. Discover herbs and spices; if you like a bit of salt, try some of the Himalayan or mineral salts available – you only need a hint to bring out the amazing flavours in meat, fish and vegetables. If you have ever made a curry from scratch, you will know that the process of adding the spices is almost like alchemy: each one you add builds up a layer of flavour that can only be described as mystical! Try getting a specific spice mix from a specialist (*see* Suppliers) or buy them separately and grind your own blend. I promise you it will beat any jar of curry sauce hands down. Herbs are a delicious way of adding subtle tastes to a dish; not only can you buy them dried, but if you have a garden or even a window box, you can grow your own. Nothing beats snipping off a few sprigs of parsley or basil from your own plants and tossing them straight into a simmering sauce on the stove – the scent is heavenly. The Hobo Packets in our recipe section just beg for a handful of herbs, so get growing! Other great additions to your condiments are soy sauce, olive oil and balsamic or wine vinegars, all of which can be used to create subtle or striking flavours to a variety of dishes.

Sweeteners – every now and then we want a little bit of sweetness, and so a jar of raw honey or agave syrup is the perfect way to get the taste, but with a bit of goodness added. Honey is an astonishing food and, when eaten in moderation, has an enormity of health benefits as well as tasting delicious. Use it sparingly in recipes that call for sugar or where you want a hint of sweetness, such as in your porridge or to take the tartness from stewed apple. Another excellent sugar alternative is stevia, a by-product of a leaf, which used to be quite hard to buy, but is now available as a calorie-free sweetener that you use as you would sugar – the manufacturers state that a sachet provides the same sweetness as one teaspoon of sugar.

Extras – things like sugar-free jam, sugar-free peanut butter, etc., are all fine to have around, but do use them in moderation.

The fridge

In a Zen Diet fridge, you will expect to find fresh meat, fish, vegetables, salad, olives, organic skimmed milk and small amounts of other dairy such as Parmesan cheese. Fresh fruit juice is fine, but drink it in moderation as it is surprising how many calories you can stack up with a large glass of juice. Fill a 250ml glass with half juice, half water. Plain live yogurt and kefir are brilliant additions to your daily diet.

Kefir is a fermented milk drink from the northern Caucasus region of eastern Russia. It is prepared by culturing a mix of yeast and bacteria known as kefir grains in milk, and kefir has been scientifically proven to benefit the gastrointestinal tract and the immune system by penetrating the intestinal lining, thereby improving the 'housekeeping' of the gut and helping the body become resistant to pathogens. It contains strains of friendly bacteria, including *Lactobacillus caucasus*, *Acetobacter* species and *Streptococcus* species. Whereas yogurt has friendly transient bacteria that can help keep the gut clean and provides a source of food for the bacteria that live there, kefir's yeasts *Saccharomyces kefir* and *Torula kefir* can actually colonize and create a system of defence. Making kefir is easy; you can obtain a starter culture from a variety of online suppliers (*see* Supplier section), and one sachet of starter can be used for up to six batches of kefir. Add the sachet to a litre of room-temperature organic cow's, sheep's or goat's milk and leave for 24 hours to ferment. It makes a curdled, runny yogurt-like drink which you can use on its own or blend into a smoothie (*see* Recipes) or you can add it to muesli or granola for a nutritious breakfast. Once it has fermented, put it in the fridge, it should keep for five to six days; you can then start another batch by using 100ml of the kefir added to your milk using the same process as before.

The freezer

Have lots of good-quality meat, fish and vegetables, but dump the ice cream and ready meals. If you want a quick meal from frozen, make a double batch of pasta sauce or stew and freeze some for later or bag some wholesome home-made soups that you can easily reheat. Instead of ice cream make your own delicious frozen yogurt – it's so simple: just fill a freezer-proof tub with plain yogurt, add chopped-up or pureed fruit, stir and place in the freezer – a quick, nutritious snack or after-dinner dessert.

Now you have sorted your kitchen, you need to tackle the art of 'eating out' Zen-style!

Eating out, eating smart

ZEN TIP

Studies in the US have shown that using a bigger fork can help reduce your food intake! When using a fork 20 per cent larger than normal, the intake of food overall was less.[1]

When you are trying to lose weight, eating out is a big challenge, mainly because studies have shown that the restaurants offering the most food, and indeed the highest-calorie foods, get the most customers. I myself have found it is very hard to manage the conflict between wanting to get value for money and the urge to lose weight. What we see as value for money is being measured in calorific terms; basically, we feel that the more calories we get, the better deal we have, which is the exact opposite of what we are trying to achieve. The truth of the matter is that, unfortunately, when dining out it's difficult to make sure you're eating the right foods. This is because most of the factors are outside your control. You don't know what kind of oils they're using to cook food or make the sauces. You don't know what kind of seasonings are being added or in what quantities, but you can bet there's a lot of salt!

Because profit drives the recipe, the food is probably not of the highest quality and it may not be fresh. The reality is that we don't want to purchase extra fat or get heart disease, but something is inbuilt: we feel terrible going to an all-you-can-eat buffet and only having one helping. Likewise we feel it is a terrible thing to buy a salad for the same price that we could have had a steak and chips. When eating out, we need to be aware that the whole world is set up against us; everything in that environment is arranged to make us eat more and to take in the most calories. It is rare that you will find a chef cutting the cream or fat in anything you eat. Often it is better to order the salad option, than to fight through the calorific nightmare that is the standard restaurant. At some places you can get your whole daily calorific intake in one single meal.

When out on the town, it is also extremely hard to keep down the calories. So, for example, you drink a pint of beer, you may as well be eating a slice or two of bread; the calories are about the same, but the damage to the body is more so. However, most people wouldn't see four or five pints as overly excessive on a Saturday night or for their birthday, and the same people would think you were slightly mad if you sat there and consumed five to ten slices of bread in one go! The other problem with drinking is that it loosens your discipline and you often find yourself eating something you didn't plan to.

So what can we eat whilst we are out and how do we avoid getting caught out?

1. The most powerful tool in your arsenal is the salad bar – if you can go somewhere that offers an unlimited salad bar, where you can have as much as you like, then you can fill up on salad – that way, you won't be able to eat as much. However, be aware that some restaurant chains' idea of salads is pasta, potatoes and such like

smothered in mayonnaise and oils. You should avoid this and stick to the main vegetable part of the bar, such as lots of lettuce, tomatoes, beetroot and the other usual salad ingredients. Use only a small amount of dressing and steer clear of the creamy-looking sauces and dressings.

2. Drinks – water of any variety, diet cola or lime and soda. Many of us have used fruit juices as an alternative to alcoholic drinks only to realize that they often contain the same, if not more, calories due to the high level of fruit sugar as opposed to the sugar contained in wine or beer. Drinks are often the easiest way to put on fat as they are easy to consume and cause your blood sugar to spike quickly.

3. One other important point to remember is to request exactly what you want – it may cause some discomfort, but if you want to lose weight or eat healthily, then you need to avoid food that has been anywhere near a deep-fat fryer, such as chips or fried rice. If the dish you want comes with chips or anything else fried, request plain boiled rice or new potatoes – if they can't do that, then ask for some of the available vegetables to be added instead. Always remember that you are paying for the meal YOU want. I have not had a problem so far getting an alternative to go with my steak, but I have seen a heated argument between a bodybuilder and a waiter when the former asked for an egg-white omelette! There are limits to what most restaurants will do.

4. Ask about condiments – your best-laid plans can be destroyed by the sauce. Remember you are living in a fat-fuel obsessed world where every restaurant or fast-food joint is catering for people with an urge for fat, and when you order your steak and salad, it often comes drenched in a creamy sauce, which has more calories than the whole thing put together. So, if in doubt, leave it out. It's not worth that one moment of ill discipline and indulgence; indeed, these exceptions that we make for ourselves are a means by which our habits are broken – the exceptions will become the rule, so focus on permanently making good food choices. When eating out, more than any other time, addict's logic comes into play. There's a reason why in this circum-stance you should change all the rules you are applying to yourself – it's somebody's birthday or some other special event, or you deserve it or you don't eat out that much – whatever the environment is you need to reward yourself or celebrate by doing what's good and healthy for you for your long-term health and happi-ness. Also, be aware the cheaper the meal, as a general rule, the higher the calories! Be prepared to spend a little more to get less fat!

5. Don't start with a starter – period – unless you are having the starter as your main, which is a great idea to keep down your calories. However, most starters are loaded with fat – usually deep-fried and not particularly nutri-tious. They call them 'appetizers', but you don't need

it; have a nice main meal and savour every mouthful instead of devouring courses for the sake of it.

6. Ditch the dessert – after a big main meal, do you really need a dessert? Ok, maybe *need* is the wrong word as no one needs dessert. You may want one, but chances are you are about to load another 300–500 calories on top of your meal. If you really want dessert, then you may need to cut a deal with yourself – you'll have salad and chicken breast at a reasonable 350 calories and then a simple dessert of, say, fruit and ice cream or sorbet.

You will have already gathered that one of the big problems with eating out is you don't know where or what. You don't know where the food is sourced, whether it came out of a packet, or indeed what's in it. Even if you do ask, it may be that because it is reheated or cooked by someone else, the person doesn't give you the correct information. This is one of the few times that standardization is good. We tend to think of fast-food places as being a negative influence on our dietary aims, but, in the case of some leading fast-food chains, this is not so. Because they clearly display the calories in every one of the meals, you can control your calories and have a meal without fear of eating too much. For example, if you have a burger, a garden salad and a diet cola, that's around 500 calories which isn't too bad for a meal, especially for a healthy adult male who weighs over 100 pounds; but likewise you can have a fish burger and a diet cola and know exactly what you are getting.

It is interesting to see that other fast-food chains are moving in this direction, and once you know the calorific values of the various meals on offer, you can start to make an educated choice which allows you to keep things under your control. In this sense, going to a non-standardized restaurant is more risky. I recently went to a wonderful Italian place in Covent Garden for breakfast and asked for scrambled eggs on toast. The meal that appeared was spectacular: it included scrambled eggs on toast, bubble and squeak, sausages, bacon and baked beans! Once it had appeared, it was far too wonderful to resist. Sometimes, going somewhere where things are less passionately produced can be more in line with our goals, even if it does not have the personal touch that other restaurants can offer.

It's amazing what small changes can have a big effect in the long term. Studies have shown that people who eat from smaller plates eat 20 per cent less than those who eat from a standard 12"-diameter plate. Our perception of how much food we have is influenced by how big the container is. Another interesting study shows that eating with your left hand decreases food intake significantly. The psychologists conducting the study believe that this isn't due to the difficulty of eating with the left hand, but rather by using the non-dominant hand, we make it a more conscious task and we stop 'automatic' eating. This is something significant to remember: most of our eating habits are absolutely automatic; we eat the same things day after day, year after year. To change that, we need to focus on making a conscious act of eating. Much of this can be done by preplanning. One study showed that people who preplanned any section of the restaurant menu, and indeed the restaurant they ate in, managed to keep to their diet far better than those who went in with good intentions. So one thing you can do is to just choose your meal from the salad section of any menu placed before you; if you only look at the salad section, you won't be tempted by anything else.

ZEN TIP

Ladies! If you want to eat less, eat with men – some studies have shown that women instinctively eat less when with a member of the opposite sex!

One final note on eating out or on the go: I find that planning snacks or planning my lunch when I'm out is ultimately the best thing to do – I might pack a salad, some chicken breast and a pint of milk. Something that is the right nutritional or calorific amount for you and your goal will also be good for your pocket as well.

ZEN TIP

Ban the bread basket! And not just the bread – the corn chips and salsa, the crisps, peanuts and any other little bowl of nibbles that we all absentmindedly pick at when they are conveniently placed before us. But it all adds up calorie-wise. If you really need something to keep the hunger pangs at bay when waiting for your meal, ask for some crudités, i.e. carrot, celery or cucumber sticks.

Holidays

A natural extension of eating out is eating when on holiday – it is a challenge. A real challenge! You may be in another country and you might not be able to self-cater. The control you have over your food is significantly reduced. When we relax, we tend to treat ourselves. If you have an all-inclusive package, it is hard not to try to get your money's worth. I think I must be the only person in the world to go on an all-inclusive holiday and not to drink a single alcoholic drink! But how can we have such discipline on holiday and how can we use our time away to burn extra calories?

I used to struggle with keeping the weight off on holiday, but over the years I have perfected the formula! First of all, I make sure I keep to my exercise routine no matter what, and with the additional calories burned from exploring and swimming, I can burn more calories than when I am stuck at work. Because the meals are so big at most restaurants, I cut out all snacks and I am very careful not to overeat. Standardization is not something I would normally recommend – it is an unsustainable tactic usually, but you don't need to sustain it, you are only on holiday for a couple of weeks!

Breakfast

On most holidays you will have a breakfast buffet. I love cooked breakfasts and used to find myself unable to resist a full English cooked breakfast every morning, but I had to find a way of preventing this. After all, a full English can have well over 1,000 calories! Basically, nowadays I have a compromise. I have a nice big bowl of fruit and then either an omelette or scrambled egg. And lots of tea! Again, I am using bulk as my ally. If you eat a full bowl of fruit, it is far harder to fill up on anything else, and it makes a great start to the day. When you are on holiday, find a high-bulk food to start with; don't think of it as an either/or. Have a low-calorie, healthy, bulky start to your meal like some grapefruit or melon and eat lots of it. Then move on to a treat of an egg or that sweet something. Just so you don't feel deprived!

Lunch

You need to have one light meal every day. I tend to choose lunch because it's easier to eat light when on the go. I tend to buy a can of tuna and a salad, and I can get this almost anywhere in the world, even in rural Japan. If I can't find that, I will buy a sandwich or the local equivalent. One warning if you are in a Middle Eastern country: avoid the falafel – they are deep-fried and calorie-laden. If you can find a salad and protein source, then you're winning. I have this almost every day for the whole period. It really helps keep the weight off.

If you *can* eat your light meal in the evening, it is far better for fat burning (more on this later). I find this quite difficult when staying in a hotel as I end up eating in a restaurant where it is hard to eat lighter food.

Dinner

You are going to have to eat out at some point, so you have to apply all the rules and tactics listed previously. When in a foreign restaurant, you may have a problem recognizing what you are ordering or knowing how it is going to be cooked. There may be few healthy options to choose from. I recommend you find what you want, or rather find the closest option, and to ask for exactly *how* you want it. Most restaurants will do what you want with no quibble.

I go to Egypt often, where steak is inexpensive, but it is frequently served with chips and other fried things. So I always ask for steak, rice and vegetables If they won't do it, I will go elsewhere! Once I find somewhere that will give me a healthy meal (like fish tagine with couscous), that's what I will eat every single evening. That's not to say I won't try the odd local dish now and again, but only one that's not deep-fried. If you can find a healthy local dish, stick to that instead. Once you find a formula that's working, stick to it.

One other tip – there are many ways to relax. Make your holiday the one that is in line with your goals. Do something active. So many people just lie in the sun drinking beer. It's an amazing planet, why not explore? You will be surprised how many calories you burn seeing it!

Snacking as an art form

Planned snacks

Snacking is important! The more you spread out your calories, the less likely you are to store any of them as fat. You see, fat storage is triggered by your blood sugars reaching a peak; if you keep your blood sugar constant, then you should decrease the probability of fat storage. Likewise, if you eat every three hours or so, you will hardly ever feel hungry and you are less likely to give in to a craving for an unhealthy meal or to overeat at a meal time.

But what to have and how to plan it? I always have something high in protein as I find that it takes a long time to digest and cuts out my hunger. You could have a chicken breast or a protein bar. I sometimes have a pint of skimmed milk or a packet of beef jerky. If you prefer carbohydrates, you need to have something that takes a long time to digest, such as rye bread or wholewheat rusks. If you are a creature of pure virtue and self-control, or if you really like vegetables, then carrots and celery or fruit are the best snacks in the world. You would have to eat a wheelbarrow of them to make a dent in your calorific input. Find something that's high-bulk and low-calorie and make sure you plan ahead and pack your snacks in the morning. To fail to plan is to plan to fail.

What to drink

Drinking is a powerful tool in your weight-loss arsenal. Studies show that those who drink more water have less body fat than those who remain dehydrated, and there are many reasons for this.

- Water makes you feel full. One study by scientists in Virginia proved that those who drank a couple of glasses of water before their meals ate a lot less than those who had not tanked up – up to five pounds less over a three-month period.[2] This is probably due to the fact that the stomach is full of calorie-free water! So drink lots, drink often, as it keeps you feeling full.

- Energy levels. It takes only a 5 per cent reduction in hydration levels to give you a whopping 50 per cent reduction in energy levels! Many people misinterpret the low energy levels as low blood sugar and decide it is time for a snack. Keep your energy levels up by staying hydrated.

- Energy release. Although there is no firm evidence, some experts believe that when you are fully hydrated, it is easier to release fat stores and that a dehydrated body goes into a conservation mode that prevents any fat loss.

- A taste of the cold. Yes, it is only a small thing, but imagine how it adds up over a few years. If you drink cold water with ice, your body has to use energy to warm you up. This burns calories and thus fat. If you can go for the cool option, have ice and lemon with your water and watch your fat melt with the ice cubes.

Protecting your motivation

It's a strange thing. When you change your life and make an effort, many people don't like it. Even when people say words of support, sometimes they are less than helpful in their actions. I think this is because many people feel inferior and disempowered when someone starts doing what they can't. For this reason you need to protect your goals and your enthusiasm from the negative thoughts of others. The world around you needs to be adjusted for you to make permanent changes. Most of us would agree that it would be hard for a smoker to give up if he lived with smokers and continued to spend his time in the places he used to smoke. We would never advise an alcoholic to keep going out with his drinking buddies if he really wanted to turn over a new leaf.

The same is true of all habits and lifestyle changes; if you want to change your life, it is best to change your habits. I, for example, used to go to an all-you-can-eat buffet with my friends every Saturday. Every week I used to kid myself into thinking I was not going to eat more than I needed. I would drink diet cola and try my best to keep down the calories, but … I always failed. The truth is that if you want to be slim, you can't keep going to the all-you-can-eat.

When I go to the gym, I notice some people whose build never changes. It's a strange thing if you think about it.

One woman I know is always on the treadmill. I have been going to the same gym for five years, and I have never seen her lose weight or indeed get any faster on the treadmill. Something is not working, and when I talked to her, I found out quickly what it was. She exercised out of guilt, as a means to burn off calories that she had put on going out partying with her friends. That's why she always used to come in on a Monday and Friday. She was almost exercising to make room for extra calories and then to take off what she had put on. When we talked in depth about her weight-loss goals, she told me a very long story of her attempts to go out night-clubbing and to keep down the calories. First she tried just drinking rum and diet cola, then she moved on to only having white wine spritzers. She had tried everything, but after five years she had made no progress. When I suggested she give up night-clubbing completely and take up something else, she was horrified. The problem is that after decades of going out drinking and eating, she couldn't dream of a world without it. At the same time she said she would do ANYTHING to be slim. After talking it over for a while, she revealed the truth: she was scared of the friends she would lose if she stopped taking part in the activity that bonded the group. She showed me a picture of her and her friends on the town. They all looked just like her! The terrible truth is she may have been right. If she decided to break the mould and to invite her friends to a yoga club or slimming group, or even to go out swimming, they would be rather taken aback. It may even be that they would start to reject her after a month of her no-partying policy!

But this is part of the path of change. It could be that she could start a revolution and turn all her friends into health buffs. However, more often than not people who have bad habits want you to stay with them and are hurt when you try to make a change. Every week I still see the same woman at the gym. She never seems happy because she is living in conflict. Remember that old saying: 'If you chase two hares, you don't catch either!' She feels bad at the gym due to guilt from the extra calories drunk the night before and feels bad when out drinking due to the effect on her health and weight. It's time for her to take a risk and move on; if her friends are genuine, then they will stay with her. If they fade away, she will need to replace her activities with something positive that puts her in touch with people who are supportive of her goals.

But how do we get in this state? We need to cultivate our goals. We need to protect our dreams and to build our hopes with a gentle effort every day. To do this, we have to make sure that we focus on far more than just ourselves; you need bigger reasons to do the things you do. You need to build your dreams and make your goals and positive motivation so strong that no one can break them down. I often practise this exercise while going to sleep or when I have a moment or two to myself on the bus or train. I find that if I formalize it, it becomes rigid and lifeless. Bruce Lee used to call this exercise 'the mental charge'. He used to sit and imagine all the things he wanted to do and focus on the wonderful events in the future.

The mental charge

Take time to imagine your goals. Use recent events to aid you in building both motivation and confidence. Try to put yourself into a situation when everything makes you stronger: for example, if you have had a success and you are happy with yourself, use that as proof of the ongoing transformation in your life and personality. If you had a day when you ate your perfect diet, think about how easy it will be in the future to be able to make this the standard.

Use setbacks and negative things to your advantage. If someone called you something rude or showed doubt in your goals, imagine how wonderful it will be to prove them wrong. Try to enjoy the feeling of success when you get to the point you dream of.

Most of all, focus on your current *kaizen* change, that small change that you are introducing to your life. Think about how powerful this small change is going to be and what effects it will have on yourself and others. If you have decided to make sure that you cut out a snack you eat by routine – for example, a chocolate bar every day – and perhaps replace it with two glasses of water and a carrot, focus on this. Don't spend much time on other goals, just image how this is going to change you and your life. The extra calories you used to take in from the chocolate bar are no longer going to be part of your daily routine, so that's 250 less calories! Over a ten-day period that's 2,500 calories, which is a whole day's worth of food less! You could only cut that number of calories by fasting for a whole day. Wow, imagine how you start to see the weight slowly coming off! Imagine how others see this happen. Everyone is looking for a secret diet of slimming product, but you know the truth is in the Zen Diet, in the small and EASY change.

Reinforce to yourself how easy this change is – just one habit swapping for another. Instead of going to the canteen for a coffee and a chocolate bar, you are going to go for a walk in your break and drink a bottle of water and have a carrot. Think of the extra calories you have burned and the health benefits of the vitamins and roughage from the vegetables. Fresh air. Imagine what others will think. Those who approve start to join you or are inspired; whereas for those who don't, use their cynicism as a strength to make the change stick and then to entertain them with another!

Really enjoy the emotions of the exercise, so that your subconscious starts to associate the small change that you are making with those positive feelings.

Now think of the example you are setting. You are making this change not just for yourself but for others around you. The people who you love and who you want to be healthy, too; perhaps you have children who you want to grow up healthy and fit. Perhaps you have a partner who you want to be as healthy as possible to enjoy life together.

Make sure the goal is as global as possible. This is your quest to stand for what you want to see in the world – health, harmony and positive focus.

Team work

'No man is an island …' as the saying goes, and this is truer about eating habits than many other things. It is not just you involved in this mission. As mentioned previously, some people will not be on your side. They will not like the change you are bringing about. This section is about those who *are* on your side. One small change you can make that is very powerful is to start to recruit help. It seems a strange idea when you first think about it, but it really is a must to have some people on your side in this mission. It's very hard to cook your children and partner sausage, chips and beans and then to make yourself a salad niçoise! So step one is to attempt to bring those close to you in line with your goal. They don't need to want to slim with you, but you just need to see if they would like to join you in making life healthier. It is far easier to go for a walk every evening with someone else than it is to go alone.

Bringing the family on your side

It's a great thing if you have someone interested in diet and health to work with you on your goal. That way, you can work together and only buy healthy food and cook the best meals for your goals. Sometimes, however, you may need to sell the idea to your partner, parents or whomever you live with. I use the term 'sell' because that's exactly what your mission is. It is best not to simply impose healthy changes on those around you (except those that they would never notice). You need to bring them on board. Don't just tell them your goals; think about what they would want from the same changes. It may be that they would like better health or to be more athletic. Look at what they want to change in their life and give them a chance to fulfil those aims. I know one woman who rather cunningly made various changes to the family diet in order to help a health complaint her husband had. By making it all about *him*, there were no complaints, and within a month he was rejecting food that he previously would have fought for!

Go to your doctor

Do go to your doctor first. He is, after all, going to be over the moon at your goals, but it is important to make sure that no existing health issues could cause problems with any of the changes you are hoping to make. But far more exciting are the ways he may be able to help you with your goal. If you are a certain weight, your area may offer a 'gym prescription' which is basically a free gym membership. They may even offer a few sessions with a personal trainer. Likewise, they may have a free slimming club or exercise group. I even know of one person who went to a doctor and came out with some lovely slimming green tea extract, all free of charge. Great result!

Slimming clubs

Slimming clubs are brilliant. Yes, they are! So many people say cynical things about them, but the truth is they work. And they replace social activity that involves consuming calories! Perfect. I know three people who have used well-known clubs and got perfect results. When you join, you instantly get a team of supportive people who have the same goal. Just remember most clubs let you carry on coming for free as long as your weight stays within your target. It's not just only for women. If you're a man and you choose to go to a slimming class, you are bound to be outnumbered, but you will get more female attention than a new baby in a retirement home for midwives. If you lack support in your goals with the people you know, a slimming club is highly recommended.

Exercise classes

If you join an exercise class, you get a new support network of health-conscious people. You also lose a bit of weight and build health every time you attend. It's a great way to gain support and have fun. However, one word of advice: I box, and as a boxer I tend to think of myself as pretty fit. One week I missed a class and decided that I should go to boxercise instead, thinking it would be easy – after all it's not *real* boxing! I was wrong. It was the most gruelling hour and a half of my life – worse than martial arts training in Japan, worse than long-distance running in the desert. Some of the exercise classes out there are very high-octane, so always start with a beginner's class or choose something gentle like yoga, aqua-aerobics, tai chi or something you really love the idea of doing. If you want to do ice climbing – do it!

Love being the most important thing, sustainability being the second. You need something you can do during the busiest, the run-down and tired stages of your life. It is better to do tai chi every week and burn an extra 100 calories than to do step aerobics twice and never go back! And remember, if you take a friend along, you are far more likely to carry on.

Obviously, there are some overweight people who find it hard to be mobile and cannot get to the gym. A gentle but persistent approach is then necessary to begin the process of not only losing some weight, but also regaining mobility in joints and muscles that have not been used properly for some time. Of course, exercise alone is not going to make you lose weight and so is just one of the small but permanent changes you need to make.

Being immobile is not confined to those who are overweight; many people have an illness or disability that also makes movement and exercise difficult, and at the back of the book is a programme of the types of exercise that can be of use to those unable to move around freely.

The gym

Some people love gyms. I love them, but not for the social side. I find it annoying when people talk to me. I am just there to exercise, and I resent anything that gets in the way of my workout. However, many people find the social side a great support. People notice if you don't come and they help you with your goals. Most gyms have free exercise classes and help you track your goals. It's a great support network if you don't have many people around you who are into health and exercise. Some individuals think of the cost of a gym as being expensive, the average price being about £25 a month. I find that those who look down on this kind of cost will spend that on a takeaway or on a night's drinking. We spend so much money investing in our car, our house and in pleasure. I don't think £25 a month is much to invest in your body.

The power of appointment

Are you ready to go for a walk? Want to go to an exercise class? Is it time for the gym?

Don't feel like going?

Going to give it a rest today, but you have a friend to pick up on the way. You can't let her down; time to get in the car. Yes, that's the power of appointment. It makes you go when you would have stayed at home. So, if you can, make sure you have a friend or two involved in everything you are aiming to do.

Peer pressure

One of the things about associating with healthy people is the power of peer pressure. It is hard to have a giant steak and chips at the vegan conference or to go to Slimming World with an ice cream for everyone! As you make new friends, you will find peer pressure starts to become your ally, rather than the alternative of people around you with unhealthy habits.

Make words match your goals and goals match your words

One study into people giving up smoking showed they were far more likely to persevere and succeed if they announced their goals to the whole universe. This seems to work on two levels. Firstly, if you say that you are a non-smoker to people around you, it starts to become part of your new sense of self. You think of yourself as a non-smoker and so you act like one. Secondly, embarrassment; none of us wants to look silly. If we have been telling everyone we don't smoke, we don't want to be caught smoking! So we would rather not smoke. The same is true with weight-loss goals. I was silly enough to post a YouTube video of myself posing and showing off my muscles before I started a new body-building regime. I said I would post my results in 60 days. A week later I realized I had to stick to what I said. I can honestly say this helped me stick to my regime.

If you are going to lose weight, be bold about it. If someone asks you about your weight, tell them that you are losing some every day. Make your goals public and invite people to share in what you do. It takes a bit of guts, but it really helps when you get to a hard point in your goals.

Small changes to food habits

The beauty of the Zen Diet is that it allows you to make big differences with small steps! Rather than radically changing your diet in one huge step (which is much harder to stick to in the long term), little steps are used to help you get used to each change before you go on to the next one. As each step becomes a natural habit, you will see a permanent change in your lifestyle and health. Each step is backed up by research and statistics proving that it is a habit worth having – there are too many diet books that give faulty or realistic advice, but here I aim to use examples and techniques that have a firm basis of success and positive health benefits.

Add some spice to your food!

Cinnamon

The delicious warming taste of cinnamon is a great way to keep your insulin at a safe level. Insulin is the hormone responsible for turning any excess sugar you consume into fat. Studies published in the *American Journal of Nutrition* showed that when volunteers were given rice pudding with 3 grams of cinnamon added, they produced less insulin after their meal. Aside from the benefit of reducing sugar levels, it may also help you feel fuller for longer by slowing down the rate at which the stomach is emptied.

Sprinkle cinnamon powder onto your food (try not to overdo it as large amounts of uncooked cinnamon may have undesirable effects[3]). The use of cinnamon supplements in capsule/tablet form may help control sugar cravings and reduce insulin sensitivity.

Cloves

The humble clove – studies[4] have shown that there may be some real benefit to using clove supplements as a way of helping reduce insulin levels in those who are diabetic or prediabetic.

Chilli

Chilli fans will be delighted to know that chilli has a beneficial effect on the metabolism. The potent ingredient capsaicin, which gives chillies their heat, is responsible for reducing hunger pangs, especially for the salty, sugary and fatty foods we need to avoid. Apparently, though, you won't get the same effect from taking chilli powder in capsule form as you do need to actually taste it.[5] You can use fresh or dried chilli as the effects should be the same.

But don't overdo it! We don't mean limit the heat, feel free to go as hot as you can stand, but studies have shown that if you only eat chillies occasionally, the appetite-curbing effect is greater.[6]

Garlic

Not only does garlic reputedly keep vampires away, but it appears to do a pretty good job at getting rid of excess weight. Trials in Israel showed that the pungent odour of garlic can help trigger the part of the brain that reduces hunger by convincing us that we are full. The main effective compound in garlic is allicin (also the stuff that gives off the smell); this has several major health benefits, including helping to prevent cardiovascular disease, improving the immune system and thinning the blood. Garlic can be enjoyed fresh or in capsule/tablet form (as long as the active ingredient allicin has been preserved – check the packet).

Five or more a day

Fruit and vegetables

As obesity becomes more and more of a problem, we have to look at what food choices we are *really* making. A lot of people believe that fruit and vegetables are expensive, but if you eat them when they are in season (more of this later), buy locally every few days for freshness, and buy just as much as you need to avoid waste, you will find that they are actually incredibly good value for money when compared to fat-laden or sugary foods. You can make some wonderfully filling, delicious and nutritious meals with just a heap of vegetables and some good-quality protein; all it takes is a bit of creativity to avoid the same old 'two veg' routine.

Eat apples

They say an apple a day keeps the doctor away, and this may indeed be true. Not only do apples have a good dose of vitamin C, an antioxidant with attitude, but they are loaded with pectin, a great source of soluble fibre that can help keep blood sugar levels on an even keel and helps lower cholesterol by binding to bile acids and drawing the cholesterol from the body.

Always eat breakfast

It looks as if Mum was right – breakfast *is* the most impor-tant meal of the day! Think about it: 'break-fast' – breaking your fast, that long, lean period overnight that needs to be addressed when you wake up. The reasoning is based on sound scientific fact. Eating breakfast, even if it is just a wholesome bowl of cereal, is a necessary requirement for your body to function healthily – on all levels. It restores those plummeted blood sugar levels and kick-starts your metabolism into its daily work. If you don't replenish your 'fuel tanks' not only do you feel empty, jittery and probably a tad grumpy, but if you don't eat anything until lunch (which is a common practice for dieters), then your body starts to go into 'famine' mode and alerts your system to start storing fat for hard times. Remember, if you skip breakfast, by the time it gets to lunch, you have potentially been running on empty for over 14 hours! This then usually leads to eating a calorie-laden lunch as your body is crying out for energy, and more often than not giving in to snacking and a heavy dinner to make up for it.

Try to eat within an hour of waking and make breakfast a protein-rich meal, with some wholegrain carbs and a large drink of hot water and lemon, green tea or decaf coffee. Try to avoid the classic 'full English' as it is way too high in fat – even though it is rich in protein. Eggs are phenomenally rich in the highest-quality protein, and having two eggs for breakfast can help reduce your calorie intake for the rest of the day.

Here are a few great, easy-to-make suggestions for getting you going in the morning:

- Scrambled egg (high in protein) on wholegrain toast – add some smoked salmon for a big boost to protein levels

- Porridge (protein/carbs) with mixed berries or honey and cinnamon

- Super Protein Shake (*see* Recipes)

- Egg-white omelette with salmon

- Wholegrain cereal with semi-skimmed milk and mixed berries

- Two boiled eggs with wholegrain toast

Sweet treats

We all like the odd sweet treat, but you can actually go for a healthy, fairly low-calorie option and still get that satisfaction normally associated with a huge sugar hit. If you are used to sugary foodstuff, at first your palate will be really disappointed and it may all seem tasteless, but the less sugar you consume, the more you will appreciate the taste of low- or sugar-free foods.

I switched to sugar-free jam years ago, and if I have 'normal' jam now which is basically half sugar, half fruit, I find it almost overwhelmingly sweet.

We talked about the health implications in Chapter 1 and also the options for using sweeteners, but one word about sweeteners – they are used massively in the food trade to replace sugar and often give us the impression we are being healthier, but there are questions about their health benefits. Some people consider them to be damaging to the health and many scares abound. The jury is still officially out on sweeteners such as aspartame and acesulphame K, but in my opinion it is better to opt for something closer to the structure of sugar such as stevia-based sweetener or xylitol or to avoid all sweeteners and sugars completely. There are lots of things you can add to food that offer sweetness naturally and in far lower quantities needed than piling sugar into them. Use honey, agave, stevia and fruit sugar sparingly and you can still have a great taste but without the calories or possible negative health consequences.

Here are a few ideas to try instead of reaching for the obvious chocolate bar.

- **Eat dark chocolate** – chocolate containing 70 per cent cocoa solids or over is a much better choice than milk chocolate. Why? Because it contains far less sugar and calories and more health-promoting antioxidant ingredients. Also, because it is far richer tasting, you don't need to eat as much to feel satisfied.

- **Dried fruit** – can be high in calories if you eat a large amount, but a few pieces of dried apricot, peach or mango can be really filling and not only satisfy your sugar craving, but also add some beneficial fibre, antioxidants and minerals to your diet.

- **No-sugar muffins** – you can make some incredibly tasty muffins and biscuits without adding sugar. Using wholewheat or spelt flour and adding dried fruit, banana or a sugar substitute such as stevia, agave syrup or xylitol, you can create something really yummy, high in fibre and low in calories. These are great for kids, too – it encourages them to have a healthy snack that doesn't taste like mushed-up cardboard. (*See* the Recipe section for ideas that include these no-sugar muffins, spelt and honey cookies and flapjacks.)

If you must snack, keep only healthy snacks in sight. According to studies, office workers snacked less when packets or dishes of sweets were removed from their desks to the other side of the room or into another room.

The same trick can be reversed to positive effect; putting healthy snacks or meals in more prominent positions can increase consumption of these healthier food items by over 250 per cent in a year.

Zen meals

Your meals are extremely important. In fact, they're the most important part of your diet. Exercise and cutting out snacks are lifestyle changes that will only go so far. The most powerful parts of anyone's diets are the three basic meals they have during the day because the majority of your nutrition comes from your main meals.

We all have routines in our meals. We have certain ones that we eat at each and every meal. We have certain ones that we eat each and every week. We all have routines in everything in life – washing, cleaning, working and sleeping. We manage our life by routine. We develop them instinctively, even if we don't notice it.

Scientists have studied people's eating habits, and most have between five and ten meals that they eat or cook in rotation each and every week. Try for yourself … make a list of all the meals that you cook and eat every week and you'll find that there's a massive overlap. There are some usual suspects that appear most weeks.

You may have a slightly wider repertoire or may have a few days where you try something new every week, but more often than not you're cooking something that you've prepared many times before. You will find that how often you eat out or get a takeaway is also part of your routine.

Analysing your routine, you'll find that some of the dishes include extremely high-calorie foods. Meals like fish and chips have up to 1,000 calories. Some kebabs have over 2,000 calories, which is your whole daily calorie requirement in one meal.

Now, imagine what an amazing change it would be by simply changing one of these high-calorie meals for something healthy and around 600 calories – meals which are far more filling than the aforementioned fish and chips or kebabs, and which have only 500–600 calories. That's why we're introducing you to *kaizen* recipes which have a lot of bulk and a lot of flavour, but are low in calories.

The good news is that all you need to do is to try them. If you find a meal that you like, simply introduce it into your diet. That way, you've made a *kaizen* change. Every time you have that meal, it's replacing one that would be high in calories. The meals are high in nutrition and amazingly filling, but low in fat and calories. In fact, I designed these meals for myself when I was practising *kaizen* for my diet.

Low-calorie drinks that cultivate health

You may have noticed that much of the Zen Diet is focused on what you drink. This is because in the modern Western diet a lot of our calories are from sugary drinks and alcohol. The problem is that these calories come in a super-easy-to-digest form, so the body converts them directly to fat!

When fruit squash and fizzy pop were first invented they were treats. Most people only had them on special occasions. Nowadays, they are everywhere in restaurants, supermarkets, petrol stations and served as the default beverage in fast-food stores. Figures from the American National Center for Health Statistics report that 50 per cent of the American population over the age of 2 consumes sugary drinks every single day. This includes sodas, fruit squash, sweetened waters, and energy, sports and fruit beverages. The report states that drinking sugary drinks is linked to 'poor diet quality, weight gain, obesity and, in adults, type 2 diabetes'.

Still fancy a free refill?

Most people get about 252 to 273 calories every day from various drinks! Imagine how these extra calories add up and how many pounds of fat these drinks could add every year! Often we don't think of the calories in the drinks we have. It is a subtle vice that provides only empty calories, and it takes the place of more nutritious options.

In this section, I am going to suggest some alternative forms of drink that feed the health, not the belly fat! But remember: if in doubt, stick to calorie-free drinks like water, sparkling water, teas and herbal infusions.

Aloe vera juice

With this aloe vera juice recipe you can make your own drink. It is simple, cheap and requires only aloe vera leaves from your own garden. Making home-made aloe vera juice is much healthier because you get the pure potential right from the plant. Commercial aloe vera products have some chemical additives to keep them stable and prolong their shelf life; therefore, they cannot be considered 100 per cent natural.

It is always better to consume the natural product if possible. So having your own aloe vera plant, you can make your own products. Home-made aloe vera juice should not be kept longer than a week in the refrigerator; don't make more than you will consume in two days.

For a normal dosage of 300 grams of pure aloe vera juice you will need approximately 400 grams of leaves from a mature plant:

- Cut the ends off the leaf and the edges.

- Split the leaf in two halves and scrape the clear gel out of the peelings. Be careful not to contaminate your gel with the latex of the leaf – this is the bitter yellow juice coming out of the peelings.

- Put the aloe vera gel in a blender, add the juice of 3 to 5 oranges or any other kind of citrus fruit and blend it for about 2 minutes.

- After blending, put it in the refrigerator to let it settle for at least 2 hours.

- After this period of time it is ready to be consumed. You can dilute this nutrient-rich drink with water or any kind of natural fruit juice to enhance the taste.

Lemon balm tea

Lemon balm is a fragrant, flavoursome herb. Simply pour hot water on the leaves to make a delicious herb tea with an intense lemon taste. So strong is the flavour of lemon balm that it is still used commercially to flavour sweets and ice cream. It is easy to grow: just plant some and it will grow in huge clumps all over the garden – remember to drink lots of it as a tea or your garden may become overrun!

In addition to being a wonderful, calorie-free and inexpensive drink there are health benefits. One study demonstrated that lemon balm helped reduce the fat levels in mice. It also has antibiotic and antiviral properties and a mild, calming effect due to rosmarinic acid contained in the leaf.[7] Far better than paying for lemon squash!

Green tea

Green tea is reputed to speed up the metabolism and has other potential health benefits. According to the *American Journal of Nutrition*, drinking three to six cups of green tea a day is purported to speed up the metabolism to burn cellular energy by up to 40 per cent more, whilst also increasing the rate of fat burning. The magic bullet in green tea is a number of compounds called catechins, the most active of which is epigallocatechin or EGCG. These catechins are believed to have beneficial effects not only on fat burning but also on reducing inflammation in the body, helping prevent cardiovascular disease, cancer and other illnesses.

Green tea is also high in bioflavonoids and antioxidants which add to the weight-loss and health benefits. Antioxidants are thought to have an effect on leptin, the protein responsible for regulating the amount of fat laid down in the body. Green tea can be drunk hot or cold and comes in various forms: teabags, a concentrated powder and also capsules.

Water

Simply drinking a 200ml glass or two of water 5–10 minutes before a meal can significantly reduce the amount you eat, effectively by just filling you up. Some studies have shown that people lost a remarkable 2 kg or more over 12 weeks by drinking water before meals as opposed to those purely on a low-calorie diet (and drinking no extra water).

Lemon juice

Another remarkably simple way to make a change is to add a squeeze of fresh lemon juice to your food or in a glass of hot or cold water. Lemon is brimming with health-giving properties and contains vitamin C, acids and pectin. All these have been shown to help with losing weight. Vitamin C helps burn fat more efficiently, with studies showing a 30 per cent increase in fat burning during exercise for those with higher levels of vitamin C in their bodies.[8] Lemon juice is known as a tonic for the liver, which plays a pivotal role in the natural detoxing of the body; it can also aid the liver by producing more bile which is a crucial part of the digestive process.

The white stuff

Milk is a great supplement to a healthy diet, but can also add a significant amount of calories – if you love a glass of cold milk, keep it skimmed and at a sensible 250mls which gives you 80 calories and a whopping third of your daily calcium intake.

Fruit juice

Not all fruit juice is as healthy as manufacturers would have us believe; many of the so-called healthy 'juice drinks' are loaded with sugar, and some haven't even been near a piece of fruit, being synthetically produced using flavourings. Even fruit juice, fresh or from concentrate, is still packed with fruit sugar and should really be viewed as a 'serving' of food rather than as a drink. A 200ml glass of fresh juice can hold up to 100 calories. As part of your normal healthy diet, either have a small glass between meals, water it down 50/50 or make a super-juice blend to have as part of your meal.

Chapter Three

CHANGES TO LIFESTYLE

THIS IS AN UNDERRATED BUT vitally important part of any 'diet'; there are so many things other than food that can sabotage your good intentions and even stop the benefits of your efforts. The Zen Diet is a holistic approach and offers advice on simple but important areas of your lifestyle that could make a huge difference to your wellbeing. All techniques and examples are proven to help with many aspects of general lifestyle and healthy living, the majority being backed up with scientific research.

Rest

Rest is as important as sleep. Most athletes know the importance of rest and recovery between activities, to maintain their physical equilibrium. What most people don't realize is that we need rest and recovery to maintain our mental equilibrium too. The sheer amount of information flooding into our unconscious every day causes our minds to be constantly on the alert, which also means that we can become mentally drained very quickly. The trick is to employ the method of 'mindfulness' once again – to rest fully you need to calm the mind, to stop the endless chatter and become absorbed in the moment. Remember when you were a child and could stare at the clouds for hours or watch a bug in the grass? Well, you need to relearn that very state and allow yourself a regular break from a hectic world.

Sleep and weight loss

Creating good sleep 'hygiene' is as important as having good physical hygiene. Sleep is often one of the most neglected areas of people's lives and yet is probably one of the main pillars of our health. Studies and surveys conducted by the National Sleep Foundation (NSF) over the last decade showed that 'at least 40 million Americans suffer from over 70 different sleep disorders and 60 percent of adults report having sleep problems a few nights a week or more'. Obviously, a few nights of disturbed sleep are not going to be a problem, but when it is a recurring event, or you are consistently skimping on your sleep due to work, study or partying, then the long-term effects can begin to take root. Science has shown us that chronic sleep deprivation, the building up of a sleep debt, can cause some serious metabolic changes, one of which is weight gain. This is believed to be due to the way carbohydrates are metabolized, which, in turn, affects the hormones that are in control of our eating patterns, appetite and weight.

According to the results of a two-phase study undertaken by researchers from the Kaiser Permanente Center for Health Research in Portland, USA, people who slept for less than six hours or more than eight hours a night were less likely to achieve their weight-loss targets than those who experienced between six and eight hours' sleep. It also concluded that high levels of stress had a significant effect on weight loss. The study was specifically looking at the association between stress and sleep and the effect it had on successful weight loss, showing that stressed people with a chronic sleep deficit were 50 per cent less successful in achieving their weight loss. This supported earlier studies that had linked poor sleep to obesity.

Sleep problems alone cannot be seen as a definitive cause of weight problems, but there certainly seems to be evidence that metabolic changes occur when the body is deprived of good-quality rest and relaxation. So much occurs when we are asleep that it is crucial to maintain a good pattern of rest and relaxation. The final conclusion of the US study showed that 'chronic stress [exacerbated by lack of sleep] may trigger hormonal reactions that result in an intake of energy-dense foods, so that eating becomes a "coping behaviour" and palatable food becomes "addictive"'.[1]

Why is sleep so important?

Have you ever pulled an all-nighter? How did you feel the next day? I bet groggy, irritable, forgetful or clumsy came into it! Even after just one night without sleep, concentration becomes far more difficult, your attention span shortens considerably, and with continued sleep deprivation the part of the brain that controls our language, memory, planning and sense of time becomes severely affected and practically shuts down. Rational judgements become harder to make, and the response to critical situations is severely impaired. Although most of us aren't going to beat the world record for staying awake (currently 11 days!), we are often chronically deprived of sleep or sleep-lagged due to our hectic lifestyles. This, over a period of months or years, can add up to a recipe for ill health.

Deficient or impaired sleep can significantly affect not only your mental health but also your immune function – according to Dr Diwakar Balachandran, the director of the Sleep Center at the University of Texas, sleep deprivation causes levels of our T-Cells (responsible for good immunity) to go down and for inflammatory cytokines to increase, thus putting us at greater risk of catching colds or flu.[2]

But what happens when we sleep?

It may look as if not much is going on; we just lie down and go to sleep, right? Well, yes, but beneath that calm façade there is a huge amount happening in our body and mind.

Our natural sleep pattern has a recurring cycle of around 90–110 minutes, split into two categories known as REM (rapid eye movement) sleep and non-REM. Non-REM has a further four phases:

Stage 1 Light sleep – we are drifting off, but can be woken easily.

Stage 2 True sleep – after 10 minutes of light sleep we slip into the next phase, which lasts around 20 minutes; our heart rate and breathing has slowed – this is the largest part of our sleep pattern.

Stage 3 Deep sleep – we begin to produce 'delta' or slow brain waves; our breathing and heart are also at their slowest.

Stage 4 Deep sleep – we are at our deepest, breathing is rhythmic, and our muscles relaxed. If we are awoken during deep sleep, we often feel disorientated and confused.

REM sleep begins after approximately 70–90 minutes after going to sleep, and we have 3–5 REM periods of sleep a night. This is when the brain is at its most active and dreaming occurs. Our bodies become almost paralysed, and eye movement can be observed; breathing rates rise, as does our blood pressure. After we have a REM cycle, the whole process begins again.

However, while all this is going on, our body is incredibly busy with other metabolic processes. We all have something that is called a 'circadian rhythm', better known as 'body clock'. Find your daily rhythm here with this fun test:

http://www.bbc.co.uk/science/humanbody/sleep/crt/

How can we improve our sleep and rest habits?

We often feel that sleep should come easy and that it is a natural thing to do, but for many people it is the exact opposite. The problems can be varied:

- **Environmental** – perhaps you live on a noisy street, have noisy neighbours or young children that wake you in the night; or maybe the house is too warm, too cold or too cluttered.

- **Physical** – perhaps you suffer from chronic pain, have acid reflux or indigestion, or another illness or disability, that affects your sleep patterns.

- **Psychological** – if you suffer from anxiety or depression, this can seriously disrupt sleep.

- **Social pressure** – some people feel they will be considered 'boring' if they go to bed before midnight or that there is something they will 'miss' on TV.

There are many things you can do to improve your sleep and rest habits. Try a few of the suggestions listed on the following pages.

Avoid light at night

As mentioned previously, our bodies work to a certain schedule called the circadian rhythm; this internal body clock is in charge of regulating all the necessary processes in our bodies, including digestion, hormone production and cell renewal, which are triggered by the complicated action of chemical messages and nerve systems.

During the day and at night our body is constantly working to produce hormones that can wake us up or help us sleep. Melatonin is one of the main hormones that triggers the cycle for sleep and is created deep within the brain in the pineal gland. It is crucial for regulating our body clock and creating our sleep patterns. We can confuse our body clock and disrupt our melatonin production by actions such as travel through different time zones causing jet lag or by playing havoc with our nightly sleep patterns.

In our 21st-century life we have more things than ever to disrupt our evenings – TV, computers, mobile phones and continual electric light. Our grandparents or great-grandparents would not have had these obstacles to sleep, and often they still have better sleep habits than younger generations. Go back 100 years and they had none of these things; if you lived in the country, you would probably go to bed by 9 pm and be up when the sun rose. Your life would have been lit by the sun or by soft light from candles, oil or gas lamps.

Today we have light at the flick of a switch, which,

although useful, has caused havoc with our nightly sleep cycles. Melatonin production ceases when the brain perceives there to be enough light; so instead of the gradual going down of the sun to dictate the evening unwinding, we have glaring light that tricks our brain into thinking it is still day, and so melatonin production decreases. Studies have shown that this has a profound effect on our bodies and sleep cycles and has caused the multitude of sleep problems we now have. When mice were subjected to sleeping under light, they gained 50 per cent more weight than those kept in darkness. Even something as simple as watching TV, checking your emails or text messages last thing or having a light on in the bedroom at night can wreck your sleep – all these things give out light. Even a crack of light through the curtains is enough to disrupt that precious melatonin production, and through continual disruption with these seemingly innocuous habits, we create sleep problems. Here are some simple ways to prevent melatonin disruption:

- Stop working and turn off the TV, computer (iPad, etc) and mobile phone at least one hour before you intend to sleep.

- Lower the lights during the evening – use softer side-lighting.

- Try not to check the time with a light if you wake up.

- Don't have a TV on standby or a lighted clock in the bedroom.

- Try to avoid turning the light on to go to the bathroom or have a soft night-light in the hall.

- Don't sleep with a light on.

Create a bedtime routine

When we were little children, the chances are we had a specific bedtime and wake-up time. As we got older, things changed: due to social commitments, work, lack of routine and peer pressure, our bedtimes probably became more erratic, and waking up depended on whether we had school or work, or if it was the weekend. But research has shown that monkeying with your sleeping and waking times can create havoc with your body and mind, causing a state similar to jet lag.

Due to our bodies' inbuilt rhythms and regular release of chemicals from the brain, to make the best of our sleep patterns and to keep ourselves healthy, one of the most important things we can do is to work out our natural sleep–wake cycle. Try to naturally identify when you start to get sleepy in the evening and then, rather than pushing through it, get ready for bed. Within a few weeks of keeping to this bedtime, you should start to see a regular waking pattern with or without an alarm clock; if you can do it without an alarm, all the better.

Avoid the temptation to sleep in at weekends as you will disrupt your natural body clock and feel groggy. There will of course be times when you need to be up later at night, but it is consistency that is the key; just go back to your usual bedtime the next day. Having a regular sleep cycle will not only benefit your mind and body, but you will often find that you are more productive with your time.

Zen your bedroom

To create the perfect environment for sleep, you need to make some simple adjustments:

- Make sure that your bedroom is neither too warm nor too cold. Body temperature is crucial to deep, healthy sleep, and it is better to be cooler than too hot in bed. Use cotton bed linen and a duvet that is adaptable for summer and winter. Try not to have the central heating on all night – it is drying to the airways and can interrupt your sleep. If your room is chilly, keep the heating on the lowest setting.

- Use blackout curtain liners or a blind to keep light out.

- If sound is a problem, try thick curtains, double/triple glazing or, if you are able, relocate your bedroom to a quieter part of the house.

- Choose a good bed, mattress and pillows – you spend a huge amount of time asleep during your life; buy the best you can afford. Some people are often happy to buy a large and expensive TV, but sleep on a dreadful bed; get your priorities right if you are one of them – your health is more important than HD TV.

- On the subject of TVs – ban them from the bedroom. The last thing you need before sleep is a mental injection of action films, doom-laden news or just plain rubbish. If you want entertainment in the bedroom, read a slow-paced book or make love.

- Keep clutter to a minimum – it is hard to relax if you are surrounded by junk.

- Use pleasant scents to help you relax; some essential oils are perfect for helping you wind down – try lavender, neroli or sandalwood.

- Allow some fresh air into your room; a stuffy room can make sleep uncomfortable.

Have a bath

Since melatonin production increases and adrenaline decreases as the body temperature drops at night, one way to hasten this is to have a warm bath before bed. As you cool down after your bath, you will begin to feel sleepy. Having a lower body temperature improves the chance of deeper sleep; after around 5 am, your temperature rises and adrenaline increases, which accordingly begins the process of waking.

Have a warm drink

It's true, your granny was right: a warm drink can help you sleep. A cup of hot water or skimmed milk can really relax you; the milk contains tryptophan, an amino acid that aids sleep and relaxation.

Avoid alcohol

Some people insist that a 'tipple' sends them off to sleep – which is fine if it is just a tipple! Alcohol can certainly help you doze off, but too much and it disrupts your sleep by waking you later. If you want a drink, have it early evening.

Avoid caffeine

Pretty obvious really – for those who like coffee, tea or cola and have trouble sleeping, the answer is simple: cut down or at least have the last cup before 4 pm. Anything after that time is liable to disrupt sleep.

Celebrations

Don't use special occasions as an excuse to go crazy with food

Just because it is Christmas, Easter, your daughter's birthday, *your* birthday, your annual two-week holiday or BBQ summer, don't use this as an excuse to throw all your good work to the wind! You can still have some great food and drink, but why overindulge?

It's easy to think 'Oh well, I'll make it my New Year's resolution to lose all the weight I've put on' or 'The diet starts tomorrow!', but statistics show that *less than 5 per cent* of those who make resolutions actually make them a permanent change! By the time three weeks have passed, unless you have cast-iron willpower, so have all the good intentions. So why doesn't it work? Part of the problem is that we often make the resolutions weeks before the actual event of New Year's Day – it is the classic 'putting things off until tomorrow'. Everything seems so achievable when it is in the future, doesn't it?

We have great visions of clearing out our fridge and cupboards and filling them with only healthy foods; we have a mental image of ourselves going to the gym every day and being able to squeeze into our new slinky clothes for the new season; but when it comes to the actual reality, what goes wrong? The problem is that inevitably we over-estimate our goal and we make it unworkable – too much, too fast. We expect immediate results and then get disappointed and demoralized when things don't materialize the way we imagined they would. This is where the Zen Diet is different. As you already have read, *kaizen* is the art of making 'small but permanent changes', and this applies to *everything* you do.

Make it easier on yourself: instead of making that list that says you *must* go to the gym every day; you *must* give up sugar; you *must* lose 2 stone; try rephrasing it and resizing it to make those changes a gradual but permanent habit. Do your best to go to the gym, but if you can't for any reason, try and fit in something active that you can do instead, such as walk home from work or vacuum the house for 15 minutes when you get in. It doesn't have to be cast in stone, but as long as you make a small change in your behaviour, it will begin to make a small change in your body. If you want to cut out sugar or caffeine, don't go cold turkey immediately as it can give you a 'withdrawal' headache or other niggles. Cut down instead: have two cups of coffee a day instead of four; have half a spoonful of sugar in your drink instead of a full one, then a quarter, and so on, until you have none. You'll find that by making these smaller changes your body will be less likely to hassle you into craving the offending food or drink and you won't notice the difference much anyway. Soon you'll wonder how on earth you used to have sugar in your tea – yuck!

There is also a huge amount of social and media hype to follow New Year's resolutions or 'get bikini-ready' for your holidays, but this is a sort of binge mentality in itself. The Zen Diet is a constant, and if you continue to make those small, permanent changes all year, then you are not buying into the idea that you can go crazy with a crash diet or two-week gym blitz and then slump back into old habits only to feel guilty afterwards and start the cycle again. The beauty of small, continual change is that very soon these things become such a part of your life that you wonder why on earth you ever considered going on a traditional diet, or why you suddenly cranked up your exercise for two weeks only to crash and burn. Imagine always being 'bikini (or trunks) -ready' and always knowing that you can control your eating because you want to and not because you have to.

So the thing to remember is to make small but permanent changes – little sacrifices that give BIG rewards!

Beware of 'feeders'

I'm sure you've experienced it: you are at a dinner party or other social function and for whatever reason you decide that evening that you aren't going to drink or have pudding, or whatever it is you want to avoid. Maybe you are sensitive to something and it always makes you feel a bit sick or upsets your tummy in other ways. You are quite happy to forgo the wine, the starter or the creamy dessert, but someone there doesn't want you to! This person, or persons, will do everything they can to make you change your mind; they will try to make you feel guilty, stupid, socially inept or other unpleasant emotions.

I am really intolerant of two things – white wine and cream; they both make me feel incredibly nauseous and have an unfortunate effect after 20 minutes that I won't go into great detail about; suffice to say that it makes me need to be in *very* close proximity to a toilet! To start with, I just thought it must be an unfortunate coincidence, but, after a few more rather embarrassing experiences of this, I realized it was not worth it. Yet I never imagined the illogical and totally negative responses I received from people. On one occasion I was offered a glass of champagne, which

I graciously refused – the initial response was hilarious, but soon bordered on insulting:

'You don't like champagne?' my hostess asked.

'No, thank you, I don't.'

'You don't like champagne?' she repeated.

'Erm, no,' I insisted, 'I really don't.'

She then proceeded to ask the same question while racheting up the incredulity along with the octave and volume of her voice. By this time I was beginning to feel a bit embarrassed as everyone was looking at me, and then she asked the billion-dollar question, 'Why *on earth* don't you *like* champagne???' Now aside from the fact that I may actually just really dislike the taste (which incidentally I do), it could be a wide range of reasons – maybe I am on medication and can't mix it with alcohol; maybe I am on a diet, maybe I am a recovering alcoholic or maybe … I JUST DON'T WANT ANY ALCOHOL!

She was so rude about it that in the end I was as graphic as I could be and told her why I didn't like or want some darn champagne. The same old scenario happens when I ask for no cream in my food. Again, I have to justify why I am not indulging; if it was celery that I couldn't have, absolutely no one would be hassling me to just try a little bit or looking at me as if I were mad. It is because cream hits the pleasure sensors for people and they can't understand how or why I would not want any; in fact, one woman I met said that she'd rather put up with the consequences than never have cream again.

But why do we need to justify why we don't want a drink or a cake or a starter? We don't, but other people want us to because, and here's the big deal, we make *them* feel bad if we aren't doing what they do. Our society is obsessed with the idea that if you don't drink, or at least don't drink until you can't stand up straight, that you are in their narrow-minded opinion some kind of ascetic dullard on a par with a monk or nun and about as much fun to be with.

Other people love to make us do what they want to do because it makes them feel better about their 'vices'; we become one of them, and to a greater extent we enable them to indulge, and vice versa. These people are called 'enablers' or 'feeders' and could be anyone from your mother, sister, brother, best friend or partner; and often we are willing participants; doesn't it always feel better when others are getting drunk together or pigging out on huge amounts of food? But they will use every approach, from the subtle such as 'Oh, go on, it's your birthday!' to the worst kind of emotional blackmail which normally involves stating how much or not you love them and they love you. We've all seen the stereotype of the 'Mama' who wants to feed up her children: they use anything from body image – 'You're all skin and bones!' – to mind games – 'You don't like your Mama's food!'

As with most human interaction, these are indicative of the subtle games in play in social or familial life. The forcing of food, drink or other substances on another is about the lack of control or discipline in the 'feeder' and is something to be avoided. If someone makes you feel bad for doing something that is beneficial to your health, mental and physical, then that is *their* problem and not yours, and is effectively a form of bullying. Don't let anyone make you feel bad for doing the right thing, but you do need discipline.

The next section follows a similar theme, but is about how we use love to get us into bad habits.

Do you bond with food?

Romantic dinners, 'date nights' and snuggling up in front of the TV with some nibbles? Quite often couples use food as a way of bonding, which is a lovely way to do it, but can become a way of overindulging on a regular basis. The emotions of love, pleasure and bonding with your mate are a potent fix of chemicals to lock you into the idea that food is the only way to do this. You certainly shouldn't avoid the odd intimate dinner together as the love benefit far outweighs the consumption of food, but only if it is a special night. The danger of using food as a means to feel close to your partner means that your brain recalibrates to equate 'pleasure' with being fuelled by high-calorie consumption that equals weight gain. Try to use these occasions for other, more intimate pursuits, and if you decide to have a sexy night in, a big meal is not going to aid this!

Keeping regular

Your digestive system is a crucial part of your body: not only does it do the most obvious job of digesting your food and eliminating waste, but it has a host of other hidden functions that can affect the way you gain or lose weight. Some people assume that the digestive system consists only of your stomach and bowels, but actually it begins at the mouth and ends … well, at your rear end! It is technically comprised of the mouth, oesophagus, stomach, small intestine, liver, gall bladder, pancreas, small intestine (including the duodenum, the jejunum and ileum), large intestine (made up of three parts, the caecum, colon and rectum), appendix and finally the anus. All these separate organs play an enormous part in dealing with our daily food intake, and it all begins in the mouth.

Even before you actually start eating, enzymes in your saliva kick off the digestive process; often the smell or anticipation of food makes the salivary glands start producing. As you chew your food, various enzymes start to break it down – amylase, which breaks down starch, and lipase which converts long-chain triglycerides into partial glycerides and fatty acids. Helped by your tongue, your food is then pushed down the oesophagus and into the stomach, where a cocktail of enzymes, acids and other processes get to work on the semisolid material.

After an hour or so, the churned-up contents are moved through to the small intestine, where the majority of digestion and absorption takes place. Bile, pancreatic juices and intestinal enzymes then work their magic to break down fats and absorb nutrients from your food and pass it into the bloodstream. Toxins and other waste are removed, to be dealt with more specifically by the liver and kidneys. What is left is then passed into the large intestine, where water is reabsorbed into the body and the fibre and other waste product moved along the bowel until it is expelled.

To help our body absorb the maximum of nutrients for optimum utilization, we need to make sure that our digestive system is a smooth-running machine. Rather than make things complicated, a couple of simple changes can make all the difference:

- Chew your food thoroughly – this allows the salivary enzymes to really begin to work.

- Eat a varied diet full of soluble and insoluble fibre (if you suffer from irritable bowel syndrome, you may find the usual sources of fibre – wheat bran, beans, pulses, etc – don't suit you, so it is probably best to include fruits, vegetables and oats in their place).

- Drink plenty of fluids.

- Sit down to eat – eating on the move can cause indigestion and wind.

- Eat regularly – erratic eating can play havoc with digestion.

- Take prebiotics and probiotics or eat plenty of live natural yogurt or kefir to help keep the natural bacteria in your gut happy.

- Try and keep relaxed – the movement of the bowel can be upset by stress and tension.

- Exercise regularly – even a brisk walk daily can help your digestion.

- Drink lemon juice in warm water – it reputedly stimulates gastric juices and aids the liver in the production of bile which is crucial to help digest food.

Making movement a regular part of your day

Sounds far too ambitious in some respects, but considering some people are sitting down for up to 12 hours a day, then the subject deserves some space. An interesting experiment by James Levine, a British scientist at the Mayo Clinic in Minnesota, showed that by keeping yourself moving throughout the day, you could reduce your risk of cardiovascular disease by up to 80 per cent. He believes that 'sitting is sort of the new smoking', and was so sure of this that he invented the 'work fit' which is a cross between a treadmill and a workstation. He encourages workers to stand whilst working or, better still, use the 'work fit' and walk while you work. His research and experiments have shown that people 'can burn up to 350 additional calories per day and perform better at work by replacing 2½ hours of sitting with standing each day'.[3]

Levine's work is based on the principle of NEAT (non-exercise activity thermogenesis) which accounts for the movement and calorie burning we can achieve in a day. Because we spend a huge amount of our time sitting – at work, commuting, watching TV, etc – we are at risk of not only obesity but a host of medical problems such as diabetes or heart disease. We also use so many labour-saving devices that our need to move around is further compromised. Statistically, in comparison to a man or woman living in an Amish community who have forsaken modern gadgets and lifestyles, we take 5,000–6,000 steps a day compared to their 14,000–18,000 steps.

So how do we make these changes?

The answer is to include as much movement into your daily routine as you can. We are not implying that you have to squeeze a daily gym session into your already hectic schedule of sitting down, but simple things like taking a 30-minute walk during your lunch break, taking the stairs rather than the lift or escalator, pacing while on the phone, housework, having standing meetings at work, cooking, standing while you talk to a friend during your coffee break, ironing or folding laundry – even fidgeting seems to be an option. You get the picture; basically, it is about moving and getting off your backside regularly throughout the day – incorporate some of these ideas into your daily life and you could burn an extra 500–1,000 calories.

Chapter Four

EXERCISE AND THE ART
OF BURNING FAT

Burning fat! That's what weight loss is all about and no one would disagree with such a statement. However, it's strange but true that very few diet plans ever deal with the issue at all. That's not the Zen Diet way! Zen teaches us a direct path to our goals; a path where we do not waver or get distracted. For this reason, it's important for you to learn to specialize in the art of burning fat. It's vital for you to understand the process of fat burning and then to learn to feel and recognize fat metabolism taking place in your own body. Approach fat burning as an art form, as you would when learning to play the piano or learning to paint. And remember: practice makes perfect.

Remember to apply the *kaizen* principles you've learned in previous chapters to your exercise. Focus on making small but permanent adjustments to your exercise routine. Once you've established that change, then, and only then, move on to making another small change in your routine.

In this chapter you will have the following *kaizen* changes to make:

- Know your enemy: understanding the mechanics of fat storage and loss

- Choose your weapon: introducing exercise to your weekly routine

- Remove habits that prevent your metabolism from burning fat

- Introduce changes that increase the after-burner effect

- Introduce supplements that increase fat burning during exercise

- Introduce pre- and post-exercise nutrition that helps burn fat

- Learn the art of resting

- Zen Meditation – adjust your expectations

Let's take a quick look at how the fat gets there in the first place.

How fat is stored

Basically fat is our body's energy reserves. It's a survival mechanism for our body to store energy in the form of fat when food and energy are plentiful so that if in the future there is a period of potential starvation, the reserves are in place.

At different times in our lives we are more predisposed to laying down fat:

- During our childhood and early adolescence

- During hormonal upheaval such as pregnancy and menopause

- In adulthood when extreme weight is gained

Women have more fat cells than men, but genetics tend to also play a role. Compared to an infant who has around 5–6 billion fat cells, a healthy adult usually has 25–30 billion; an overweight adult ranges from 75 billion to a terrifying 250–300 billion fat cells in the morbidly obese.

Fat cells can shrink or expand depending on how much 'fuel' a person takes in – think of the body like a car; the fat cells are the fuel tanks holding on to the excess fuel. When you are taking in the right amount of food (calories), the fat cells stay small, but when the calories exceed your energy output, the fat cells store up the excess and expand just like a balloon!

Fat also tends to be stored when you eat a large quantity of food at one time. Studies show that eating lots of calories in one sitting is the worst thing you can do. People who eat the same number of calories over a whole day have far lower body fat. It is a fact that you don't 'lose' fat cells; they just shrink as you maintain a healthy weight and lifestyle – if you go back to eating badly and not exercising, they will fill right up again!

ZEN TIP
To keep burning fat and keep your fat cells minimized, consume fewer calories than you burn (energy in) and exercise regularly (energy out) every day.

About burning fat

The human body draws on three forms of fuel constantly – these are carbohydrates, proteins and fats, but its preferred form of fuel is sugar. In fact, the body converts any form of carbohydrate we eat into a form of sugar called glycogen which is stored in the liver. The body constantly draws on all three sources of energy, but it takes special conditions for it to start to take the majority of its energy from fat stores. This fat-burning mode is known as *fat metabolism* or *lipolysis*.

Fat metabolism is naturally triggered in the body when it runs out of other forms of fuel, i.e. blood sugar, carbohydrates from food or that stored from previous meals in the liver in the form of glycogen. As mentioned before, your fat is your reserve tank and your body needs to be encouraged if it's going to draw on it. The only two ways of doing this are to either be starved of food so that your body doesn't have anything else to run on or to exercise so that it runs out of fuel and needs to draw on the fat stores in order to keep going.

When the body runs out of blood sugar, a complex hormonal mechanism is triggered which starts the release of fat out of your fat cells and into your bloodstream. Once you begin burning fat, you need to use up 3,500 calories to burn 1 pound (0.45 kilograms) of fat. Your aim is to create a calorie deficit of 500 calories from your diet each day, so you would lose about 1 pound a week (500 calories x 7 days = 3,500 calories). Exercise along with cutting calories helps boost your weight loss.

During every day of your life you have two wonderful opportunities to burn fat – through waking exercise and a sleeping fast. This chapter covers both these things.

Burn fat while you sleep

A big opportunity to burn fat every single day is during the night. If you sleep for eight hours, that is the longest fasting time you will experience every day. During this time you will have to draw on your fat reserves to keep your body going and it is great because you are asleep, so as long as you don't wake up, you will not feel any hunger! This is one of the most powerful fat-burning discoveries I have ever made. If you follow my advice, you will wake up every morning with slightly less fat. It is the most motivating thing in the world when you see that your waistline is shrinking every day.

How much fat you burn, however, depends on a few things: firstly, when you last ate, and secondly, what it was that you ate.

No food after 7 pm

Part of the reason I discovered the super-powerful fat-burning method was by doing the opposite. I found that if I ate a large meal at night, I would wake up with more belly fat. Yes, I had really added some overnight! With men, it seems that fat both goes on and comes off the belly quickly. Many people will tell you it is a myth that eating food late at night stores as fat, but I have found it to be completely true. One thing I do know, and is scientifically unquestionable, is that if you wish to enhance the effect of the natural sleeping fast, you don't want to go to bed having just eaten. So if you make sure the very last thing with calories that passes your lips is before 7 pm, you will find that you are burning far more fat when you sleep. Try it for two weeks and see the difference.

Low-carb dinner

This is the most powerful dietary change I have ever made. The trick is to make sure that you eat a meal that has lots of bulk and slow-release energy as it is horrible and demotivating to wake up hungry in the middle of the night. I started by having a salad every evening with little carbohydrate and lots of protein like chicken breast or tuna. Yet I found that, although this is one of the quickest ways of burning fat, it is not a permanent change I want to make. Instead, I have a routine of eating a variety of low-carb dinners – if you would like some ideas, look in the Recipes section of at the back of the book. The important thing is to make sure you have lots of vegetables and protein and keep the carbohydrates low and complex. Don't eat anything sweet at all in the evening. If you have any problems being motivated on this matter, ask yourself what you want your body to burn overnight: ice cream or your body fat.

If I have had a low-calorie evening meal, I also sometimes have some protein powder with water or some cottage cheese just before going to sleep. This makes sure I don't wake up hungry in the night and raid the fridge.

If you follow all these guidelines, then you will find that after you go to sleep, your body soon has little energy to run on. The protein will slowly release a trickle of energy and amino acids that will stop your body burning muscle, but not enough to maintain blood sugar levels. Your body will have to fire up the fat-burning enzymes to do that. With that perfect balance going on until breakfast, you will have eight to nine hours of your body constantly burning fat.

Try it for a week and wake up slimmer every day.

The perfect low-carb dinner is of course a salad; here's a section that will inspire you!

Salads

If you are looking for a healthy option, salad could be a perfect choice. It does, however, depend on what's *in* your salad. If it consists of a small amount of green vegetables covered in mayonnaise and hidden under many layers of croutons, cheese and dressing, then you are going to be loading on the calories, not burning them off. Likewise, it is hard to keep eating a salad every lunch or dinner time if they get repetitive and boring. I spent a year perfecting the art of making a salad. It's the perfect meal because you can eat as many vegetables as you like and really fill up. The best weight-loss formula I have ever found is to eat a large salad for dinner with some good complex carbohydrates and high protein. That way, I could eat as much as I liked so that I would not get hungry overnight. The only problem is it does get a bit boring. After a few days your mind rebels and starts trying anything it can to trick you into eating something else. For this reason, in order to maintain your salad focus, you need to be a master salad maker. You need to know all the slimming tricks and build your meal like a green architect.

Making the ideal salad

So you want to be able to make a healthy, filling, slimming salad at the drop of a hat and you want to be able to vary it enough that you fancy eating it every day. Variation means your body gets lots of different nutrients and it's healthy to have variety.

Here is the first and most important principle of salad building: it must be filling! Yes, the main thing is that you fill your stomach so well that you don't end up eating something more calorific in a few hours' time. Think about it in terms of 'how can I get the most salad with the least amount of calories?'

To do this, you need to make sure you have lots of vegetable bulk. The best way is to use cabbage or lots of chopped carrots or celery, peppers and cucumbers. They work really well and create a nice crunch to what you are eating.

Be creative with your salad options. You can make some delicious salads with some very interesting ingredients. It pays to spend a while each time you visit the supermarket looking at the vegetables they have. They vary more than you think. There are some interesting vegetables with strong flavours that have really low calories. Try adding some asparagus to your salad. Boost the flavour by adding Parmesan cheese or some anchovies (Parmesan is 7 calories a teaspoon) – lots of flavour but low in calories.

Use salad dressing that has low calories and high flavour; to do this, you can add ginger or garlic. If you don't want dressing, try a few slices of fresh ginger or garlic. The main thing is to use ingredients that add punch and nutrients, not excess calories. Every time I make a salad, I put in a handful of roasted salted sunflower seeds or mixed seeds, not just because it gives it a nice crunch, but it is healthier. However, the seeds are high-calorie, so don't have too many; just add enough to make it interesting.

The main key in making salads is variety, and for this reason I have included a list of possible ingredients that you can use, some of which will surprise you. Make sure you try them all.

Protein base

Decide on your protein base and then add whatever takes your fancy.

Meat – grilled chicken, steak, sliced hams, beef, chorizo (go easy as it can be high in fat)

Eggs – hard boiled

Cheese – feta, Parmesan, cottage cheese, halloumi

Fish – tuna, salmon, sardines, mackerel, anchovies

Cooked pulses/beans (canned or dried) – chickpeas, black-eyed peas, kidney beans, Puy lentils, cannellini beans, sweetcorn (fresh or frozen), green peas (fresh or frozen)

Cabbage

Cabbage is the best vegetable for salads. I always have lots of finely sliced white cabbage as it is sweet and crunchy and it fills me up for a long time. It may not taste like it, but cabbage is high in vitamin C. It is also packed with glutamine, an amino acid that has anti-inflammatory properties and helps prevent muscle breakdown. Some studies have also linked glutamine to human growth-hormone release. It's so low-calorie you can eat as much as you like. I have no idea why, but after eating cabbage my body temperature rises, so there is something thermogenic in it.

Peppers

Peppers come in different colours – red, yellow, orange and green. To liven up your salad, make sure you have a couple of different colours. I find red and yellow are the best for salads; they go well with rice-based salads or with coleslaw. You only need to eat half a pepper to get your daily recommended dose of vitamin C which helps fight against free radicals (molecules that are linked to cancer). Studies into the effects of vitamin C, conducted by Arizona State University, show that it assists in fat oxidation, or the body's ability to burn fat. So make sure you add some yummy peppers to your salad.

Broccoli

Easy to cook and delicious to eat, broccoli is a great addition to a salad. Some people enjoy it raw, but I find that a bit like eating grass; I like to cook the broccoli and add it to a rice-based salad or have it with couscous. Broccoli is known as a super-food because of its amazing nutritional content, but did you know it can reduce your blood pressure due to its high levels of potassium? According to the Mayo Clinic, researchers found that potassium dilates blood vessels, which, in turn, increases the volume processed by your kidneys, hence lowering blood pressure.

French beans

Perfect for bean salads and salad niçoise, these delicate beans are full of vitamins and minerals and add a little protein, too. Lightly boil until still a bit crunchy and then add to salad.

Tomatoes

Cherry tomatoes are the best in salads: just wash them and bung them in. But all tomatoes are really good for you as they are packed full of lycopene, vitamin A, vitamin C, vitamin K, fibre and potassium. They also add bulk and flavour. I often find that if I am not in the mood for a salad, a few tomatoes change my mind!

Avocado

This delicious fruit is packed with almost 20 essential nutrients, including vitamins C and E, B vitamins, folic acid, potassium, zinc and phosphorus. They also contain both monounsaturated and polyunsaturated fats which are crucial for helping prevent cardiovascular disease. One fifth of an avocado, or 30g, is roughly 50 calories, so is perfect for adding to salads or mashing and putting on crackers.

Celery

There is a joke that you burn more calories chewing celery than it contains; whether that is the case, it is true that celery is very low in calories at only 16 per 100g. But it is amazingly dense in nutrients and adds great flavour and crunch to a salad. Boost your intake of vitamins A, C, K (helps with bone mass and prevention of Alzheimer's), folic acid, B2, B3 – not to mention antioxidants such as zeaxanthin, lutein and beta-carotene, which are also invaluable at helping protect the body from cancer and other immune-damaging diseases. The list of benefits to celery is almost endless, and this humble vegetable should be on everyone's plate.

Carrots

A great high-vitamin bulky vegetable. I like to grate two or three carrots into each of my salads. I used to chop it up, but you get a bit sick of chomping through all that bulk. Yes, it's true that vitamin A does improve vision – it is also good for bone growth and the immune system. Carrots are also low-calorie, so keep adding them to your diet to see a slimmer you.

Spinach

I love spinach, but you need young, tender spinach leaves if you want to eat them raw. The flavour can be a bit overwhelming, so don't put too much in. Be aware that it does not go with everything; try it with egg, tomato and salads with lentils.

Red chard

I had never heard of this either. I had, however, eaten it when I had bought packs of mixed salads. It's a bit like spinach, but the stalks add a lovely red colour to your salads, and it is full of nutrients.

Rocket

The Greek physician Dioscorides (*circa* AD 40–90) said that this leaf was 'a digestive and good for your belly'. Rocket is peppery, strong and very versatile; it is delicious in salads, wilted in pasta or on top of a pizza. Easy to grow all year round indoors and out, sow some rocket in a container or window box for a quick, fresh salad.

Watercress

I always feel virtuous eating watercress. I think perhaps it is because I think I will be getting different nutrients from something grown on gravel beds. It's really peppery and strong, and I am never sure if I like it or not! I am told by many that it aids in detoxing, but I have seen no evidence that any food changes the rate your body clears toxins. However, it is so rich in phytonutrients and antioxidants that it is worth adding a handful to your salad – vitamins C, K and A; not to mention calcium, beta-carotene, lutein and zeaxanthin, all of which are excellent free-radical scavengers and a powerhouse of nutrition for your eye health.

Lettuce

If you find cabbage is too heavy, then lettuce is the best thing. Once again, you want to use it for bulk, but there are lots of different types, so do experiment to find the one you like best. To me, there is little difference, but I know some people swear by one type or another.

Romaine

We have been eating this lettuce for over 5,000 years! I really like it as the leaves are thick and slightly sweet with a kind of nutty flavour.

Oak leaf (green and red varieties)

You know the one with the wibberly leaves! It's best to get this one when it's young, leave it for a few days, and it really is like eating oak leaves. It comes in both green and red varieties. Easy to prepare because it has no heart, this lettuce has a kind of earthy taste. I love it.

Frisée endive

This one looks like frilly dandelion leaves. It also tastes like them a little; it's a bit bitter with a grainy texture. Did you know it is a member of the daisy family? Anyway, it's great with poached eggs and bacon or mixed with other leaves, but don't try to use it for the main bulk of your salad as it is too bitter and may be too overwhelming.

Lamb's lettuce

I don't know why, but lots of people seem to grow this one in their gardens. It has got velvety leaves with a delicate flavour, is easy to rip apart and add to any salad; no chopping needed.

Iceberg lettuce

I think this is the king of lettuces – it is lovely, light, crisp and bulky. It's cheap and you get a lot for your money. I eat this one every day!

Onions

I always add some onions to my salad, normally spring onions, but I will use whatever we have. Sometimes they have been a bit too strong and really have blown my head off. Shallots and leeks are also nice, but spring onions are the best for salads. They also have great nutritional value with lots of vitamin C and B_6, potassium and manganese. They also contain sulphur! But don't worry, it is not of the devil! It has been linked with cardiovascular health and is believed to lower cholesterol.

Radishes

Now and again I get some radishes. I can't stand them all the time, but they add variety. They contain lots of vitamins, but also work as a digestive tonic due to containing a digestive enzyme called 'diostase'. Some studies suggest that they may also help with respiratory health.

Salad dressing

There are some good, low-fat dressings on the market although they tend to be high in sugar and salt. But there's no need to buy a salad dressing as it is easy to make your own super-healthy ones. The following recipe is the one I use almost every day:

FAULKS' DRESSING

1 dessertspoon cider vinegar
ground pepper
a dash of lemon juice
1 teaspoon of good olive oil

Put the ingredients into a small lidded jar or pot and shake them up – you can add a squirt of salad cream, some garlic, mixed herbs or mustard seeds. I promise you that with a little experimentation this salad dressing will be better than anything you could buy and with hardly any calories at all!

Adding carbs

If I have a salad during the day, I tend to use bread with my salad. I get the lowest-calorie wholewheat bread, dice it and mix it with the rest of the salad. If I am having salad for dinner, I am willing to put in more effort and tend to eat one of the following healthy carbs.

Couscous

Lots of people go on about couscous as an amazing health food. I was rather disappointed to find out it is just ground wheat! Anyway, it's nice with some herbs and spices and with some finely chopped-up salad with fish. It's amazingly easy to prepare – just pour some hot water on it and leave for 5–10 minutes.

Bulgur wheat

Richard Faulks, who is the nutritional and scientific advisor for this book was involved in a study that showed that bulgur wheat is the most slow-releasing of complex carbohydrates you can consume. This form of whole wheat is quick to cook as it is already parboiled. It is pleasantly nutty and high in fibre, B vitamins, iron, phosphorus and manganese.

Rice

You can include either brown/wholegrain rice or white basmati in your salads; both types are low in the glycaemic index, meaning they take longer to digest and don't contribute to a sugar spike. Wholegrain rice is high in complex B vitamins and amino acids and makes a good addition to your daily fibre intake. It takes longer to cook than white rice, but is worth it for the nutty taste and its filling nature.

Wild rice

Not strictly a rice but an aquatic grass native to North America; these days, it is not technically wild as it is grown on farms. It was originally deemed sacred by the Native American Indians and was collected by hand from lakes. Similar to brown rice, it takes around 45 minutes to cook in water or stock. It makes a nutritious and varied change to plain rice and is great in salads, stuffings and other dishes where you would normally use rice; you can also add wild rice to basmati or wholegrain rice.

Quinoa

Once sacred to the Incas, quinoa (pronounced kin-wa) is a nutritious and protein-dense grain, containing essential amino acids and good quantities of calcium, phosphorus and iron. It is easy to cook and just needs to be simmered for around 15 minutes. Eat hot or cold.

Nuts and seeds

Full of protein and nutrients, nuts and seeds are a simple addition to any salad, but don't add too much as they are also quite calorie-dense.

Walnuts

A classic addition to salads, these amazingly nutritious nuts will add a good dose of essential fatty acids, vitamins B_6 and B9, A, E and a host of minerals, not to mention protein and fibre. Five walnuts a day is enough to provide the daily requirement of linoleic and alpha-linolenic acid (omega-3 fatty acids), which are believed to have a positive effect on reducing inflammation in the body and protecting against heart disease.

Almonds

Almonds are high in alpha-tocopherol, a type of vitamin E, which may help reduce the risk of Alzheimer's, according to a study by the National Institute on Aging. Another study has indicated that people suffering from clinical depression have lower levels of alpha-tocopherol. Vitamin

E is also known for its ability to help repair free-radical damage. Like walnuts, almonds are rich in essential fatty acids, protein and fibre.

Cashews

Although high in calories, a few cashews sprinkled on your salad or added to a stir-fry pack big health benefits – monounsaturated fatty acids like oleic and palmitoleic acids (those that help lower bad LDL cholesterol and increase good HDL cholesterol), protein, fibre, B vitamins and a host of minerals, including zinc and selenium. Remember: a little goes a long way, but the benefits really do outweigh the odd indulgence.

Sunflower seeds

These deliciously nutty-flavoured little seeds contain a variety of nutrients, including selenium, essential fatty acids and amino acids, which are the building blocks for our bodies' growth and health. They are quite high in calories, so a small handful is adequate to provide you with a daily dose of goodness.

Pumpkin seeds

High in calories, but even higher in nutrients, these lovely crunchy seeds are a valuable addition to your diet. High in protein and amino acids, including tryptophan (which is nature's tranquillizer), these little green seeds offer a hefty dose of B vitamins, minerals and essential fatty acids. Sprinkle some on your salads or toast them on a baking tray with sunflower seeds to make a tasty snack.

Sesame seeds

Sesame seeds have been eaten for millennia and were used in oil form by the ancient Egyptians, who were aware of their excellent nutritional value. Like the other seeds, they are high in phenolic antioxidants, which are excellent at mopping up free radicals in the body to help prevent cancer and other immune-destructive diseases. They also boast a large range of amino acids, vitamins, minerals and omega-3 fatty acids. Add a handful to your daily diet to receive your quota of these important nutrients.

Flaxseeds

Flaxseeds are full of omega-3 fatty acids, linked to reducing heart disease, Alzheimer's and depression. One tablespoon will give you 2.3 grams of this essential nutrient and also a good dose of fibre.

Exercise – choose your weapons!

It is extremely important that you choose a form of exercise to introduce to your weekly routine; it should be something you enjoy and of an intensity that you can maintain during the most busy and stressful periods of your life. It's important to approach exercise with a sense of joy. It is not a form of work, but the chance for stress relief every day – and your number-one tool for weight loss.

Exercise is by far the most efficient way of burning fat.

When the body is fasting, it burns a much higher percentage of protein or muscle. We want to maintain muscle mass because muscle burns fat all day, every day! So it is important to learn how to burn fat during exercise. But all exercise routines are not born equal. Some burn more fat than others, and it's extremely easy in a modern gym environment to work out for half an hour without burning any fat.

Signs that fat metabolism has kicked in:

- It takes 20 minutes of exercise before you turn on your fat-burning metabolism.

- A second wind – you suddenly feel that you have more energy.

- Drive after disillusion! This is a common feeling in people who are just starting an exercise regime. Before your fat starts to burn, there will be a lag, which is a period of low blood sugar when you find it hard to exercise. This is followed by an increased sense of optimism when your body switches on its fat-burning mode.

- An increase in breathing rate – as you start to burn fat, you will notice a change in your breathing rate. Some people also note a different 'feel' to their breath. This is due to more carbon dioxide in your breath as you start to burn the fat.

- A feeling of fat burn – yes, sensitive individuals report they can feel the change as their body starts to burn fat. They can feel the energy flowing into their blood stream.

So there it is: about 20 or 30 minutes into exercise you should feel a second burst of energy. Your breathing rate should increase naturally, and you may even feel a slight change in the way you are breathing. Each and every breath is burning fat as you exercise. Learn to recognize this sense of fat metabolism in exercise as it will also help you recognize it in daily life.

What type of exercise is best?

The exercise needs to be ongoing and preferably aerobic. Interestingly, the more intense the exercise, the higher percentage of muscle in your body will burn in desperation to supply energy. Studies have shown that walking is the most efficient form of exercise for burning fat. Many exercises use up more calories, but also burn a lot of muscle (which we want to keep because it keeps up our metabolism). Walking burns more fat per calorie than any other exercise. Unfortunately, you need to do a lot of walking in order to use up the calories required to shift fat. So you are best off finding a slightly more intense form of exercise that you can enjoy doing two or three times a week. However, always remember the Zen Diet principle that an enjoyable method is the best approach. If you enjoy weightlifting or a form of sport that is not aerobic, we suggest that you work towards burning about 300 calories in each of the exercise sessions. The amount of exercise you need to do to achieve this goal varies depending on what you're doing. Below is a chart that gives you general guidelines on the calorie expenditure per hour. But please don't use your activity based on being high calorie-expenditure – it is far more important to choose something you are actually motivated towards and enjoy.

Weight of person and calories burned

Activity (1-hour duration)	160 lb (73 kg)	200 lb (91 kg)	240 lb (109 kg)
Aerobics, high impact	511	637	763
Aerobics, low impact	365	455	545
Aerobics, water	292	364	436
Backpacking	511	637	763
Basketball game	584	728	872
Bicycling <10mph, leisure	292	364	436
Bowling	219	273	327
Canoeing	256	319	382
Dancing, ballroom	219	273	327
Football, touch, flag, general	584	728	872
Golfing, carrying clubs	329	410	491
Hiking	438	546	654
Ice skating	511	637	763

table continues overleaf

	160 lb (73 kg)	200 lb (91 kg)	240 lb (109 kg)
Activity (1-hour duration)			
Jogging, 5mph	584	728	872
Racquetball, casual, general	511	637	763
Rollerblading	913	1,138	1,363
Rope jumping	730	910	1,090
Rowing, stationary	511	637	763
Running, 8mph	986	1,229	1,472
Skiing, cross-country	511	637	763
Skiing, downhill	365	455	545
Skiing, water	438	546	654
Softball or baseball	365	455	545
Stair treadmill	657	819	981
Swimming, laps	511	637	763
Taekwondo	730	910	1,090
Tai Chi	292	364	436
Tennis, singles	584	728	872
Volleyball	292	364	436
Walking, 2mph	183	228	273
Walking, 3.5mph	277	346	414
Weightlifting	219	273	327

How hard should I exercise?

Research shows that fat is burned when you exercise at 70–80 per cent of your maximum heart rate. This can be an extremely hard thing to measure when you're working out in the gym, so scientists have come up with a simple solution that you can use to make sure you're exercising at the correct level of intensity to burn fat.

ZEN TIP

Always exercise so that you could have a conversation with the person you are next to. This is known as the 'talk test'. If you find you are so out of breath you can't conduct a reasonable conversation with a person on the treadmill to the left, then you are burning precious muscle instead of body fat.

So that's the intensity sorted. But how long should you exercise for? As with all things, you should remember *kaizen* in your exercise. Little change! If you are new to exercise, you should start extremely gently. I would suggest that if you have not exercised for a while, then you should only spend five minutes on your first session and work up by one minute each time. Other exercise authorities would find this a rather ludicrous suggestion, but they don't understand the value of small change. I have personally seen so many people boom and bust with exercise routines by overdoing it and trying to keep up with more experienced individuals.

When you undertake a new exercise routine, your body needs time to adjust. Lots of extremely complex things are happening in your bones, your muscles and in your blood vessels. Your body is learning to produce enzymes that burn fat and growing new blood vessels to distribute energy more efficiently to the areas you're exercising. In addition, your muscles are becoming better at resisting lactic acid and growing stronger; your bones are gaining increased density and adapting their internal structure to what you are doing. The art of exercise truly is the art of hinting to your body to make this change. Writing as an extremely experienced exercise enthusiast, I can truly state that the biggest form of setback is when your exercise routine injures you! Exercise should never cause any pain or discomfort to your body or your joints; if it does, you need to approach it more gently. Always remember *kaizen*! Make progress slowly.

Things that stop fat metabolism

One of your next changes may be to remove some of the things you're doing that could be causing you to prevent fat metabolism when exercising. Here are the most common culprits.

Sports drinks

Whatever you do, don't drink sports drinks. A lot of people arrive at the gym and buy sports drinks to keep them going through their session. The problem is that the standard sports drink contains 395 calories, and so an average person running at 8mph for half an hour will burn only 300 calories. Worse still, because they are continually sipping on the sports drink during their exercise, they never will trigger fat metabolism. Then, after their exercise routine, they probably feel that they can reward themselves with a protein bar or a treat on the way home. The net result is that there is no fat metabolism at all!

Alcohol

When people start a diet, they focus on cutting calories and they switch to a light beer option or start drinking slim-line tonics with spirits. The truth is it's time to let go of the alcohol completely. It's not the calories that are the problem: it's the alcohol itself.

- The moment you drink some alcohol, you stop the fat-burning process dead. It's the first fuel of choice for your body, so the moment it hits the bloodstream, your body converts straight over to 'running' on the alcohol.

- Alcohol stimulates the appetite with cravings for unhealthy foods – pizza and kebabs at 3 am … enough said!

- Alcohol also has some unhelpful effects on the body, the first being to lower your testosterone and raise your cortisol levels. A single night of drinking raises levels of the muscle-wasting hormone cortisol and decreases muscle-boosting testosterone for up to 24 hours!

Testosterone, which has a powerful fat-loss effect, is reduced whenever alcohol is consumed, and when levels are lowered, it may even lead to muscle loss. Muscle, as you will read later, is in fact the slimmer's best friend!

Reward eating after exercise

This one can sneak up on the best of us! When we exercise, we feel we have done something virtuous; we also believe there is some form of negative calorie bank and that we can treat ourselves straight afterwards or in our next few meals. The truth is, it's very easy to eat far more as a reward than you have burnt through exercising. Fish and chips or a big curry can put on over 1,500 calories – which is the equivalent of six hours' walking!

Muscle building

Be aware that no matter what form of exercise you start, it is likely that, to begin with, your weight will start to increase. This may seem counterintuitive, but is, in fact, an extremely good sign. Muscle weighs over four times more than fat. As you start to exercise, your body will begin to adapt by increasing the amount of muscle you have and creating new blood vessels to aid in the circulation of nutrients and body.

But why do we want to put on muscle? Well, muscle burns fat constantly. It requires calories to maintain muscle, so it burns out your fat stores every moment of the day;

for this reason, protecting your muscle is an important principle in fat burning.

Pre- and post-workout nutrition

Studies have shown that the way you eat immediately before and after a workout is important with regards to the kind of results you get from your exercise. Participants who took a protein supplement both before and after exercise were approaching a 90 per cent more efficient fat-burning rate and built far more muscle. Most surprisingly of all, this is a more significant effect than that of the overall nutrition during the day. So make sure you drink a protein-rich drink like a glass of milk before and after your exercise. It may seem strange to eat more calories to burn more calories, but the payoff is significant (almost doubling your results).

After-burn effect

It is good to be aware that you don't stop burning calories as soon as you stop exercising. Your body is revved up and your metabolism is in high gear. Basically, you continue to burn calories up to 20 minutes after each exercise session. Studies show that a small amount of caffeine increases the amount of fat burned in this period, so have a nice cup of tea!

The actual number of calories burned after exercise depends on how high the intensity of the exercise was in the first place. Studies suggest that there is a significant increase in after-burn when you exercise in intense bursts rather than a session of continual gentle exercise.

Because of the after-burn effect, it is also more efficient to divide your exercise into two rather than one large session: for example, if you normally spend 40 minutes on the treadmill, it may be more efficient to burn fat if you divide your exercise into two 20-minute sessions.

The power of the after-burn effect is highly individual. Some people burn lots of calories after exercise, and some don't. You will have to experiment to find out how effective this is for you.

ZEN TIP

All our bodies are different; experiment with different forms of exercise routines to find what works for you. And remember – measure results with a tape measure, not with a set of scales.

Supplements that can help fat metabolism

Yes, the stories you hear are true! There are forms of supplements you can take which do increase the amount of fat you burn during your exercise. These are extremely powerful because they optimize the fat-burning effects of the exercise you are already doing. These supplements are collectively known as 'thermogenics' because they increase your body temperature and quicken your metabolism which will burn more calories during exercise.

Here are some of the best known thermogenics:

Caffeine

This well-known substance is a useful thermogenic found in tea, coffee, cocoa and the South American plant guarana, and has long been considered an aid for improving physical performance and associated fat burning. Athletes often use caffeine to enhance their endurance powers and race performance, but it is also of benefit during short intense exercise such as weight training.

Due to caffeine's fat-burning ability, there has been much interest in whether it actually does promote fat loss. Research over the past few decades has shown that consuming caffeine before exercise enhances fat burning during actual exercise by around 30 per cent as well as increasing calories burned after exercise.

ZEN TIP

Consume 100–300mg of caffeine in the morning and an hour before training.

Green tea

Currently it is hard to find a fat-burning product that doesn't include green tea extract because recent research studies have confirmed that green tea in standardized doses can significantly aid fat loss. Green tea contains catechins, one of which is a substance called EGCC (epigallocatechin gallate), and it is this compound that is responsible for the main fat-loss benefits. EGCG inhibits an enzyme that breaks down norepinephrine – the neurotransmitter that aids in regulating metabolic rate and fat burning.

ZEN TIP

Drinking green tea is good (as it has other excellent health-boosting properties), but for optimum fat-burning benefits take a supplement three times a day before meals, containing 500–1,000mg of standardized green tea extract. Research has shown that the body absorbs catechins from the standardized extract more efficiently than from the tea.

Forskolin

Forskolin is the active chemical derived from the herb *Coleus forskohlii* (a member of the mint family) and has been clinically proven to enhance fat loss and boost testosterone levels in men.

ZEN TIP

Supplement with 20–50mg of forskolin two or three times daily before meals.

Carnitine

Carnitine is an amino acid that has been clinically proven to boost fat burning and bolster testosterone. It transports fat for efficient burning, improves fat loss during exercise and aids muscle growth and recovery.

ZEN TIP
1–3 grams of carnitine in the form of L-carnitine, acetyl-L-carnitine or L-carnitine L-tartrate with breakfast, pre- and post-workout meals and the evening meal.

Bitter orange

Synephrine is the active ingredient in the plant *Citrus aurantium* (also known as bitter orange). Chemically it is very similar to ephedrine (which is now banned), but it boosts the metabolism without dangerously elevating the heart rate or blood pressure. Synephrine works by stimulating the breakdown and release of fat, raising metabolic rate and reducing appetite.

ZEN TIP
To achieve benefits, take 200–600mg of standardized *C. aurantium* or 5–20mg of synephrine, two or three times per day before meals.

It is a fact that most gimmicky slimming tablets are constructed of the above ingredients. While thermogenics can be effective, they can also be stimulating, so don't take them less than 2 hours before bed time.

How to measure your progress

During your Zen diet transformation, it's vital that you keep motivated and that you can see yourself progressing. It is great to learn to enjoy gentle progress and to celebrate every little change you see. How you feel and how you look are the two most important pointers. I find that each time I find a genuine improvement to my diet, I notice a change in my energy levels and thought processes and even a change to my eyesight! However, fat loss is one of the most important and enjoyable side effects of a correct diet, so how do we keep track of that?

Should we use the weighing scales? But muscle weighs more than fat and your weight can change depending on how dehydrated you are at the time. How do we find out if we have lost fat?

Body fat calipers

Body fat calipers are the perfect tool for keeping track of your body fat. Calipers have been proven to be far more accurate than any of the body fat scales and as precise as underwater or hydrostatic weighing, which is expensive, inconvenient and often time-consuming. So body fat calipers are fantastic, low-cost, portable devices that you can use at your own convenience with no cost per use.

The calipers measure how much subcutaneous fat (fat under the skin) a person has by pinching a skin fold just above the hip. You then put the measurement into an equation to show body density and body fat percentage; this gives you an estimation of your body fat.

One thing to note, however, is that no form of fat measurement is 100 per cent accurate. Whatever method you use, there is room for error; even hydrostatic weighing is only accurate to within 2–3 per cent. All things considered, you should be looking at the big picture. Don't get too worked up by a small change in your reading. It is important to use the right equation for the calipers you purchase. Instructions are included in the pack and you should focus on using the same calipers and the same equation if possible. After all there are over 100 equations you could use.

One thing you may note is that the chart supplied asks you to line up your age with your fat measurement; this is because young people store about one half of their body fat under the skin. As we age, a greater proportion of our body fat is stored internally. This means that skin-fold measurements for a young and old person have different meanings; they might have the same measurement, but their body fat percentage would still be considerably different. Obviously, there are more differences than just age; gender, fitness level and race all play a role. Most equations take a few of these into consideration.

All this aside, using body fat calipers as a way to determine body fat percentage gives you amazing accuracy to within 4 per cent. That's far better than any scales. If all this sounds a bit complicated, you can do what I do and not use any equation at all! I don't even try and convert skin folds into a body fat percentage. Instead, I just note down the skin-fold measurements and monitor their change over time – simple. As long as the skin fold is getting smaller, I know I am winning.

If you really do want to have a number for body fat percentage, then just use it as a benchmark for progress. But be careful if you start comparing it with your friend who was tested by a different person or on a different system.

Always use the same spot

This is another key technique for using body fat calipers! Always make sure that you measure from the same spot. No matter how detailed the diagrams are in the instruction manual, a few centimetres make a huge difference.

How can you overcome this problem? When you read your instructions, they will give you a location to take the reading. This is normally over one of the hip bones, but there are systems that work on other sites: for example, some systems use the abdomen skin fold site which is 1 inch to the right of the belly button. Whatever option they are choosing to use, make sure you measure it with a ruler, don't guess. If they say the triceps site is midway between the tip of your shoulder and your elbow, use a ruler to measure exactly halfway; that way, you can see exactly how you are doing.

Trust me, testing your body fat with calipers may seem a bit complicated, but once you get the hang of it, it's the most motivating thing to be able to see your body fat slowly drift away with every passing week. Watching such progress in a material way is one of the keys to the kingdom. Without that, it is hard to keep a focus or indeed to enjoy the whole thing.

A note on spot reduction

In the 1980s, it was quite popular to promote the idea that you could reduce a certain amount of fat from one area of the body specifically by focusing on exercising that area. Studies during the early 1990s disproved this theory by showing that body fat reduction appeared to come in a genetically pre-set order when individuals were given different forms of exercise.

However, more recently studies into blood flow to fat tissue have modified our opinion again on spot reduction. It is now conclusively proven that if you exercise your legs, you will indeed draw slightly more energy from fat reserves on your thighs, but the majority of your fat will be burned from your major fat stores – the level of fat drawn on the specific body areas is actually extremely small. Spot reduction does have one important purpose – motivation! It's an extremely motivating thought to know that when exercising a body part, you are, in fact, encouraging fat to be burned around the exercised area.

ZEN TIP

Keep yourself motivated by imagining the fat burning from the areas you're exercising. Imagine the fat being drawn out into the blood stream and burnt as energy.

Back to burning – how much and where?

By introducing the positive changes brought in the Zen Diet, you will start to see a change in the amount of body fat you are storing. Observing this is one of the most motivating things in the entire world. But how much fat are you likely to lose and from where will it go first? The Zen Diet is designed to create small but permanent changes to your habits which will result in a deficiency of about 100 calories a day. This, in turn, will result in losing a pound of body fat with very little loss of muscle each and every week. The areas that tend to lose fat first vary from person to person, and, as a general rule, you will be able to see it come off first where it went on last.

Men and women vary in their fat-loss patterns. Men, for example, tend to have a 'quick on, quick off' rule with fat. Women tend to have a hard slog shifting belly fat, and it is only when it has come off from their buttocks and hips that it starts to disappear from their mid-section.

Rest and recovery after exercising

A Zen master in Japan once said to me, 'The start of discipline is with rest and recovery.' This is something that he had learnt the truth of over the years. You must make sure that as you introduce increased physical activity into your life that you have adequate rest and relaxation. The three pillars of your exercise routine are – exercise, nutrition and rest. Make sure that your sleep and your downtime is sacred and that you give yourself adequate recovery.

Without rest the body will not respond very well to exercise and you will be at risk of injury. A tired mind will find it very hard to keep to any discipline. Earlier on in the chapter we talked about the negative habit of eating as a form of reward. Rest on the other hand is a beautiful positive reward for exercise and something that you should cultivate.

Zen meditation – exercise expectations

It is important to be aware of what is achievable for an average person with an average lifestyle. If you are looking for washboard abs, you may be surprised at what form of sacrifices and unhealthy things you need to do to achieve this. The people you see in photographs are often models who are willing to go through all sorts of unhealthy practices to get themselves into that condition. Male models, for example, often don't drink any water in the whole day prior to their photo shoot so that their abdominals show. I know of female models and professional wrestlers who only eat two low-carbohydrate meals a day in order to achieve their physique. These extremely unhealthy practices generate equally unhealthy expectations in what forms of changes we can make in our body. The Zen Diet is about making a healthy positive change to yourself. To achieve physical form that you see on many professional actresses and models you need to skim off so much body fat that it only consists of 10 per cent of your body's total mass, which is about the same as a marathon runner. And as you can see from the photographs in many glossy magazines, these women with extremely low body fat have mysteriously managed to maintain one of the largest fat masses on their body – namely their breasts. In these cases this is always achieved by two silicone supplements!

Train to be a slim, beautiful and healthy you and let go of the foolish images projected to you in the media. We all have our own bodies and our own talents. We can't all aspire to extremely genetically predisposed individual standards.

Find a place of natural beauty away from where you will be disturbed. It could be a beautiful lake or other natural place: perhaps in some woods where you can sit and watch the wildlife. Take a few moments to let your breathing naturally slow down and relax the whole of your body. Look at the beauty around you and see how gentle everything is. Notice how the areas of life in balance are the most beautiful, whereas areas of destruction, when things are out of balance, become eyesores.

Contemplate on the beauty of nature and how it is linked to balance. Notice how nothing is extreme – everything is in its own natural perfect order. Look at the animals in the fields or the birds flying above you; observe their natural beauty. See how in animals of the same species there is some significant variation in each animal, but note how all seems to have equal beauty and grace.

Now bring these principles back to yourself. Close your eyes and visualize yourself in your ideal form; imagine how the balance brought into your life by your exercise regime is going to bring you to your natural healthy physique. Really visualize this perfect you. And when you feel ready, take a moment to step into the picture in your mind's eye and become that image. Know that you take this image with you in your daily life. Carry it in your mind; in your body is a program or template as to where your path is going to take you.

NOTES

Chapter 1 – Mental Changes
1 University College London Phillippa Lally, http://www.ucl.ac.uk/
   hbrc/diet/lallyp.html accessed 1/1/12
2 http://zenhabits.net/

Chapter 2 – Dietary Changes
1 *Readers Digest*, October 2011, p115
2 ibid
3 http://www.medicalnewstoday.com/releases/41026.php accessed
   23/09/11
4 ibid
5 Ludy, MJ, Mattes, RD, *Physiology & Behavior*, Vol 102 (3–4),
   pp251–8, March 2011. Epub 18 Nov 2010. 'The effects of
   hedonically acceptable red pepper doses on thermogenesis and
   appetite.' Abstract available on http://www.ncbi.nlm.nih.gov/
   pubmed/21093467
6 ibid
7 Yoon, M, and Kim, MY, *Pharmaceutical Biology*, Vol 49 (6), pp614–19,
   'The anti-angiogenic herbal composition Ob-X from Morus alba,

Melissa officinalis, and Artemisia capillaris regulates obesity in genetically obese ob/ob mice'. Abstract available on http://www.ncbi.nlm.nih.gov/pubmed/21554004

8   Johnson, Carol S, *Journal of the American College of Nutrition*, Vol 24 (3), pp158–65, 'Strategies for Healthy Weight Loss: From Vitamin C to the Glycemic Response'. Abstract available on http://www.jacn.org/content/24/3/158.full (accessed 7/03/2012)

Chapter 3 – Changes to Lifestyle

1   Elder, C R, Gullion, C M, Funk, K L, DeBar, L L, Lindberg N M & Stevens, V J, *International Journal of Obesity*, 'Impact of sleep, screen time, depression and stress on weight change in the intensive weight loss phase of the LIFE study', Vol 36, pp86–92, Jan 2012 Summary available on http://www.nature.com/ijo/journal/vaop/ncurrent/full/ijo201160a.html (accessed 9/1/12)

2   Mann, Denise, article on WebMD website entitled 'Can Better Sleep Mean Catching Fewer Colds?' Available on http://www.webmd.com/sleep-disorders/excessive-sleepiness-10/immune-system-lack-of-sleep (accessed 7/3/12)

3   Bankston, Amanda, writing for the Minneapolis *Star Tribune*, article entitled 'Office-dwellers stand up to 'sitting disease'', January 2012. Available on http://www.knoxnews.com/news/2012/feb/09/off-the-couch-active-options-feb-10/?print=1 (accessed 8/3/12)

APPENDIX ONE:
WEEKLY ROUTINES

IN THIS SECTION WE GIVE some suggested *kaizen* schedules that allow you to make changes in a synergistic order. That is to say, the changes work together and each one builds on the other so that they are stronger than the sum of their parts. We have made sure that each change improves on the next and builds into a fat-burning force. Remember that the changes you are making are ones you want to continue for a lifetime. When we start a new diet, we tend to be very motivated and want to introduce many changes at once. So you may find yourself wanting to rush ahead and introduce many changes immediately because you are motivated towards change. But keep your powder dry! We want to make sure that these changes are permanent, so take a week to make sure that they become part of your being.

A Ten-Week Course

This is the basic routine of habit transformation. It is set up with some powerful changes at the start, which will quickly start the fat-burning process. This will build motivation and get things moving. Remember: your fat-burning response is trainable and does get better as time goes on. With each week that goes by, everything starts to progress. Every week your body starts to burn more fat and change shape. You will be amazed to see what progress you can make with just ten small changes.

Optimum schedule

Week	Zen Change	Page
1	Low-carb dinner	151
2	No food after 7 pm	151
3	Introduce a Zen recipe every day	196
4	Exercise	166
5	Cut out all calorific drinks	118
6	Waste, not waist	27
7	Get the health-freak buzz	12
8	Planned snacks	97
9	Add in fat-burning supplements	176
10	Cut out use of lifts and other labour-saving devices	144

A spiritual approach to weight loss

Many people who have bought this book have done so because they are looking for a method that solves the problem at source and offers a more balanced, life-changing approach to weight loss. This schedule is for those people.

Week	Zen Change	Page
1	Manage your expectations	62
2	Meditation	50
3	Mindfulness	36
4	Cultivate contentment	23
5	Detachment	65
6	Waste, not waist	27
7	Get the health-freak buzz	12
8	Baby tigers	68
9	Half-day fasting once a week	
10	Full-day fasting once a week	

A routine for very rapid weight loss

This is a very strict routine that gets the fat burning at high speed. It's really only for those who have great skill in changing their habits or are very motivated to make a change. Remember that the routine means these changes are for life.

Week	Zen Change	Page
1	Exercise routine	166
2	Introduce a Zen recipe every day	196
3	No food after 7 pm	151
4	Cut out all calorific drinks	118
5	Low-carb dinner	151
6	Get the health-freak buzz	12
7	Waste, not waist	27
8	Cut out use of lifts and other labour-saving devices	144
9	Eat only Zen snacks	222
10	Eat soup or salad for lunch	153
		210

A schedule for those unable to exercise

Week	Zen Change	Page
1	Plan rewards	63
2	Inform those around you of your goals	109
3	Join a slimming club or online group	106
4	Get the health-freak buzz	12
5	Auto-suggestion	40
6	Waste, not waist	27
7	No food after 7 pm	151
8	Cut out all calorific drinks	118
9	Introduce a Zen recipe every day	196
10	Low-carb dinner	151

Your choice

You may of course wish to put together your own course/s to follow from the advice you have gained from the book, and so we have included a blank table below for your own use, to photocopy and use as much as you wish. You are the best person to plan your change as you are aware of your lifestyle and of the areas that you can change with most effect. Remember to plan a reward for each change you introduce and to keep motivated. Don't stop making changes after ten weeks, but carry on fine-tuning your diet until you are totally happy with your weight and health.

Week	Zen Change	Page
1		
2		
3		
4		
5		
6		
7		
8		
9		
10		

APPENDIX TWO:
ZEN RECIPES

In THIS SECTION WE HAVE a selection of simple yet nutritious recipes that can complement your Zen Diet. They are low-fat, nutrient-dense and simple and quick to prepare. We have deliberately not included a calorie-counted weekly plan as that is not what is needed – the 'small but permanent change' method means that you can choose your own dietary plan, but with the knowledge you will have gained from this book, it means that you make the right choices. Don't forget that Chapter 4 has an extensive section on building salads with a range of inter-esting ingredients.

SUPER-NUTRITIOUS BREAKFASTS

People on diets often think that skipping breakfast or having a very small one is a way to aid their weight loss. In fact, it is probably the worst thing you can do. You have just been literally fasting for anywhere between 7–10 hours, and your body has been going through its nightly repair and natural detox process; the first thing you need to do is replenish your energy by levelling your blood sugar levels with something totally nutritious and, crucially, a breakfast that is filling. One problem with our heavily processed and carbohydrate-rich Western diets is that they create inflammation in the body. This causes a whole host of problems from hormonal imbalance to insulin resistance which, in turn, contributes to weight gain. Choosing simple foods that help reduce inflammation is the way to go, and the breakfasts that follow are perfect choices.

SALMON AND EGGS

Really simple and quick is to scramble 2 eggs and serve with 50–100 g wild Alaskan salmon (canned, freshly grilled or smoked) – a perfect combination. If you need an extra boost of energy, try a slice of rye or spelt bread with some olive oil spread or a small amount of organic butter.

OATS AND BERRIES

Make a simple porridge from 50 g oats, 250 ml of organic semi/skimmed milk. While the porridge is simmering, add a handful of fresh or frozen berries: blueberries, raspberries, blackberries or whatever you like. If you really need some sweetness, add a teaspoon of manuka or raw honey and/or a sprinkle of cinnamon. Delicious!

KEFIR SMOOTHIE

½ pint/240 ml kefir
A handful of fresh/frozen fruit or berries – can be anything from mango, banana, strawberries, raspberries, blueberries, etc
1 small tsp manuka honey or agave syrup (optional, depending on if you find the kefir too sour)

Put all ingredients in a blender and whizz until blended.

BREAKFAST SHAKES

The best breakfast I have ever found in terms of nutrition is the breakfast shake – a milkshake with all the ingredients of a good breakfast included. In fact, I find that with a breakfast shake I eat far more healthily – there is no way I would get that many fruit, herbs and multigrains normally. It's a low-calorie and easy-to-absorb boost to the day as soon as you wake up. I guarantee that as soon as you shift your breakfasts to shakes, you will start to feel a distinct improvement in your energy levels, health and adaptive control. Put all ingredients into a blender, blend and pour into a cup.

THE ROYAL MINT – DESIGNED TO AID FAT BURNING

- ½ pint/240 ml skimmed milk
- 1 tsp of flaxseeds
- 4–5 mint leaves
- 2 ice cubes
- 2 scoops chocolate whey protein
- 2 oz/50 g oats

Put all ingredients into a blender, blend and pour into a cup.

THE AMAZING HULK – GET UP AND GO

This is a mild, green nutritious shake with nerve-feeding and slimming benefits. Pecans have strong antioxidant qualities and have been clinically proven to reduce cholesterol and to aid in weight loss due to a metabolic boosting effect. They also work as an appetite suppressant.

2 scoops vanilla protein
2 oz/50 g unsalted pistachio nuts
1 mint leaf or 1 drop of peppermint extract
½ pint/240 ml cold water or low-fat milk
3–5 ice cubes

Put all ingredients into blender, blend and pour into a cup. This tastes great without the mint, so don't worry if you don't have any. The shake is a light green even without food colouring, but if you want it green (like 'The Hulk'), you'll need a few drops.

BERRIES & CREAM

This is my standard breakfast shake. I vary the fruit but always make sure I load up on the protein powder to make the whole thing nice and thick. Be careful not to overdo it or you will end up eating the whole thing with a spoon.

2 to 3 scoops vanilla or chocolate whey protein

2 oz/50 g oats

1–2 handfuls mixed frozen/fresh berries

1 pint/480 ml skimmed milk

Optional extras

2 tsp of good-quality cocoa powder

1 tsp creatine monohydrate powder

1 tsp glutamine powder

1 tsp flaxseeds

1 tsp coconut butter

Put all ingredients into a blender, blend and pour into a cup.

SUPER-CHARGED ENERGY SHAKE

½ pint/240 ml skimmed milk

1 heaped tbsp peanut butter (or a handful of
   mixed nuts)

3 scoops chocolate whey protein

2 oz/50 g oats

1 tsp strong instant coffee

Optional extras

2 dessertspoons of flaxseeds

1 tsp of glutamine powder

1 tbsp creatine powder

1 oz/25 g mixed seeds

Put all ingredients into a blender, blend and pour into a cup.

SUGAR PLUM SHAKE

2 scoops of vanilla protein powder

1 or 2 pitted plums

1 tbsp multi-vitamin powder (*see* Suppliers section)

1 whole peeled lemon

½ pint/240 ml of water

a couple of handfuls of ice cubes

Put all ingredients into a blender, blend and pour into a cup.

VAN-ORANGE SHAKE

You either love or hate this one! Yes, it's a bit strange, but it does seem to knock your appetite out for the whole morning. Give it a go and see what you think.

2 scoops of vanilla protein powder
orange juice – to taste
a couple of handfuls of ice cubes
1 tsp vanilla extract
1 banana
a handful of frozen strawberries
1–2 tsp stevia-based sweetener

This will get your taste buds going! Put all ingredients into a blender, blend and pour into a cup.

BANANARAMA SHAKE

Nutritious and gets you going!

    2 scoops whey protein (vanilla or banana flavour)
    1 banana
    2 oz/50 g bran flakes (or your favourite breakfast cereal)
    1 pint/480 ml water
    1 tsp brown sugar
    a handful of nuts
    1 drops vanilla essence/extract
    3–4 ice cubes

Put all ingredients into a blender, blend and pour into a cup.

ALMOND EXPLOSION

Super-healthy and balanced, this meal replacement shake is so lovely it tastes like a pudding!

    2 scoops of vanilla protein
    ½ pint/240 ml of skimmed milk
    2 oz/50 g oatmeal
    2 oz/50 g raisins
    12 chopped almonds
    1 tbsp of peanut butter

Put all ingredients into a blender, blend and pour into a cup.

READY-STEADY OATMEAL SHAKE

In most of the shakes so far, when there is oatmeal, it is dry and uncooked. If you're short of time, you can use dry oatmeal or oat flour with this recipe, but it is really far better if you use cooked oats.

- 2 oz/50 g dry oatmeal, cooked in water and cooled
- 2 scoops vanilla protein
- ½ tsp cinnamon powder
- 1 tbsp chopped nuts (almond, flaxseed or peanuts also work well)
- 12 floz/350 ml water or low-fat milk

Put all ingredients into a blender, blend and pour into a cup.

SUPER SLIMMER

- ½ pint/240 ml water
- 1 tbsp flaxseed oil
- ½ ripe peach, peeled
- 6 frozen strawberries
- 1 scoop protein powder of choice
- sweetener to taste (optional)

Put all ingredients into a blender and blend.

NADA COLADA

This is a healthy twist on the non-alcoholic cocktail. Coconut oil is high in omega-3 and omega-6 oils and has great health benefits. A lovely shake if you like piña colada!

2 scoops vanilla protein powder
¼ pint/120 ml pineapple juice
¼ tsp rum extract
1 tsp coconut oil
1 packet artificial sweetener
¼ pint/120 ml water (or low-fat milk)
3–6 ice cubes

Put all ingredients into a blender and blend.

STRAWBERRY SUNRISE

I love this shake. I had it every morning for months – sometimes with some oats whizzed in, but normally with loads of fruit!

4 scoops vanilla whey protein
¼ pint/120 ml water
1 pot strawberry yogurt
lots of fresh/frozen strawberries and other berries
1 tsp creatine powder
1 tsp flaxseed oil

Put all ingredients into a blender and blend.

'GOING THE DISTANCE' SHAKE

Named in honour of the theme tune to Rocky Balboa's final fight in the film, this shake is the perfect breakfast for those about to go and hit the streets. The eggs can be raw or hard-boiled. (Just remember that raw may seem cool, but you are taking a risk of salmonella poisoning. I say cook the eggs, but it's up to you.) I have this one as a treat now and again.

   3 organic/free-range eggs (raw or boiled)
   ½ pint/240 ml milk or 3–4 scoops vanilla ice cream

Put all ingredients into a blender and mix.

PEANUT BUTTER AND BANANA SHAKE

I love this shake, but I only have it when the rest of my meals in the day are really strict. Nuts have an amazing amount of calories, so be careful. I use a small square of whole honey-comb, but a teaspoonful of honey does just as well. Don't have this every day!

2 scoops vanilla protein powder
3½ oz/100 g almond flakes or pecans
1 tbsp peanut butter
½ pint/240 ml skimmed milk
1 banana
1 tbsp honey

Put all ingredients into a blender and mix.

THE TOTAL MEAL REPLACEMENT SHAKE

This recipe is for a total meal replacement, with oats for complex carbohydrate and cottage cheese to boost the protein. You can add more milk if the mix is too thick. You can use this if you are in a hurry for a quick nutritious meal replacement. This recipe includes cottage cheese, but you won't even notice it as the blender removes the texture.

½ pint/240 ml skimmed milk
3½ oz/100 g low-fat cottage cheese
3 scoops whey protein powder (vanilla or chocolate
  works best)
1 pot low-fat, plain yogurt
1 scoop of your favourite fruit (frozen berries or
  a banana)
1 tsp stevia-based sweetener
ice cubes (optional)
2 oz/50 g dry oats

Put all ingredients into a blender and mix.

LUNCH

Lunch can be your main meal of the day or a quick but nutritious filler. Here are a few simple meals for lunch at home that only take minutes to prepare. If you are taking lunch to work, check out our salads that can be easily made up the night before. Of course, you can always swap these recipes for your supper.

SUPER-SQUASH SOUP

This is incredibly easy to make and freezes perfectly. Make up big batches that you can just reheat in 5 minutes. Squashes are also really easy to grow if you have a rough patch of land; they hardly need tending and you will be rewarded with a good harvest in the autumn.

SERVES 4
PREPARATION TIME 5–10 mins
COOKING TIME 30 mins

   1 butternut squash (or any other variety of squash) – chopped into small cubes
   2 onions – chopped
   1 yellow/red pepper – chopped roughly
   1–2 cloves garlic – chopped
   1 medium sweet potato – chopped into small cubes
   1 tbsp good olive oil

1 tsp garam masala
1 tsp turmeric (gives a gorgeous colour and subtle
   flavour)
1–2 tsp vegetable bouillon
boiling water – enough to cover the vegetables

Peel and roughly chop all the vegetables, place in a large saucepan with the olive oil and spices and allow to sweat and soften for 5–10 minutes.

Add the boiled water so that it covers the vegetables and sprinkle in the bouillon. Bring back to the boil, turn down the heat and simmer for 20 minutes or until soft.

Allow the soup to cool, then blend until smooth. Heat through before eating.

This works beautifully accompanied by some herby or cheesy bread.

SALAD NIÇOISE

A classic favourite and one that is packed with nutrition – eggs and fish provide your protein, and you get a good mix of vegetables to add bulk and taste.

SERVES 4
PREPARATION TIME 5–10 mins
COOKING TIME 10 mins

   4 oz/110 g mixed salad leaves (rocket, baby spinach, etc)
   2 cans of tuna in brine or water
   a small can/jar of anchovies (optional)
   4 hard-boiled eggs – chopped into quarters
   4 medium tomatoes – cut in quarters – or a handful of
      cherry tomatoes
   4 oz/110 g French beans (fresh or frozen) – cooked until
      tender
   10–12 baby or salad potatoes – cut into halves
   black olives

Dressing
   6 tbsp extra virgin olive oil
   2 tbsp white wine vinegar
   1 tsp Dijon mustard
   salt and ground black pepper to taste

Tear the salad leaves into pieces and place in a large serving bowl.

Drain the cans of tuna; flake and add to the salad leaves along with the cooked French beans, hard-boiled eggs, tomatoes, potatoes, olives and anchovies.

Put all the ingredients for the dressing into a small bowl and whisk thoroughly, pour over the salad and serve.

PITTA POCKETS WITH SPICY CHICKEN, MIXED PEPPERS AND BEANS

Quick and easy to make, this lunch is full of protein and fibre.

SERVES 2
PREPARATION TIME 5 mins
COOKING TIME 10 mins

  2 large pitta breads
  2 chicken breasts – diced
  1 onion
  a handful of mixed peppers – sliced
  1 can mixed beans
  1 tbsp good olive oil
  1–2 tsp chilli spice mix

In a non-stick frying pan, seal the chicken and sauté the onion and peppers.

When the chicken is cooked through, add the beans and chilli mix and fry for a further 2–3 minutes.

Scoop into the pitta and enjoy with a tomato salad.

SUPER SUPPERS

HOBO PACKETS

Hobo packets are great. It's the most convenient way of cooking you will ever discover and a great way of making low-calorie, high-nutrition food with all the convenience of packet cooking. They give you another way of eating lots of vegetables and filling up with protein. I eat them as part of my routine as evening meals, simply because I can't stand salad twice in one day. If I eat salad in the evening, I find myself awake at night. The vegetables you use in Hobo packets seem to last longer due to their high starch content.

The best thing about Hobo packets is how easy they are to make. You just get everything you need in one place, chop it all up and throw it in the oven for 40–50 minutes. Sometimes I even assemble the packets the night before, put them in the refrigerator so that in the evening I just have to turn on the oven at the appropriate hour and stick the packets in.

> *Tip:* If you choose to follow this method, let the packets warm up slightly by taking them out of the refrigerator while the oven is heating up.

Hobo packets are very versatile. They can be as simple and easy as a couple of pork loin steaks or as high-class as the lovely dish Salmon en Papillote – the basic cooking instructions are the same. Remember that the aim is to eat as many vegetables as possible so your calories remain low and you feel full up. With Hobo packets, the vegetables take on the flavour of everything added – it's a lovely warm and filling meal.

How to make a Hobo packet

1. Tear off two large pieces of cooking foil or grease-proof paper and place flat on your counter.

2. Cut up your ingredients. They need to be quite small to cook properly, so prepare thin strips of meat or bite-sized portions. You can use any type of meat, fish or fowl and add as many vegetables as you like. I also like to put in some gravy, stock, soy sauce, lemon juice or a drizzle of olive oil and then add herbs and spices.

3. Fold up the paper or foil to make a firm, water-tight packet and place on a baking tray.

4. Put it in the preheated oven at 200 degrees Celsius for 40–50 minutes or until thoroughly cooked. *Always make sure that the contents are piping hot throughout and that any meat is cooked through and juices are clear.*

5. Open, eat and then throw away the wrapper!

JUICY PORK PACKETS

SERVES 1
PREPARATION TIME 5–10 mins
COOKING TIME 40–50 mins

2–3 slices organic/freerange pork tenderloin or pork
    chops – cut into strips if preferred
1 clove garlic – finely minced
8 white button mushrooms or sliced mushrooms
2 sticks celery – diced
2 tsp dry mixed herbs or fresh thyme leaves
1 large onion – chopped as finely as possible
salt and freshly ground pepper or barbeque sauce

Follow the basic Hobo packet recipe.

CHINESE STIR-FRY CHICKEN PACKETS

This is the best Hobo packet ever. I make this at least once a week, much to my wife's irritation; she has had enough of them! It is low-calorie and low-carb, but high on flavour. I hope you like it as much as I do.

SERVES 1
PREPARATION TIME 5–10 mins
COOKING TIME 40–50 mins

- 1–2 chopped chicken breasts (seal in a frying pan first if preferred)
- 1 onion – chopped finely
- ½ each red, yellow and green peppers – cut into strips
- ½ can sweetcorn or 5 whole baby sweetcorn
- soy sauce, rice vinegar, sweet chilli sauce
- 2 tsp toasted sesame oil

Dress the chicken, onion, peppers and sweetcorn with soy sauce, rice vinegar, sweet chilli sauce and a very small amount of toasted sesame oil. Wrap in foil and bake as before.

TROUT PACKET

This is a lovely Hobo packet – great for a romantic meal. Use one fish per person and stuff it with any vegetables you like. The ones listed are an example, but anything goes with this one.

SERVES 2
PREPARATION TIME 5–10 mins
COOKING TIME 40–50 mins

   2 whole gutted trout
   1 sweet potato
   1 courgette
   a handful of green beans (fresh or frozen)
   1 onion
   2 large tomatoes or a handful of cherry tomatoes
   a splash of olive oil
   juice of half a freshly squeezed lemon
   herbs and spices to taste

Wrap in foil and bake as before.

SALMON AND NOODLES WITH MIXED VEGETABLES

SERVES 2
PREPARATION TIME 5–10 mins
COOKING TIME 10–20 mins

- 2 salmon fillets
- 1 tbsp sesame oil
- 1 inch/2 cm of fresh ginger, finely chopped (optional)
- 1 garlic clove – finely chopped
- 4–5 tbsp soy sauce
- 6 spring onions – finely chopped
- ½ red pepper – sliced
- ½ yellow pepper – sliced
- 1 medium onion – thinly sliced
- 2 nests of egg noodles or a pack of ready-to-wok noodles
- 1 tsp black sesame seeds

Steam or pan-fry the salmon (if steaming, this will add to the cooking time by approx 15 minutes).

Heat the sesame oil in a pan and fry the ginger, garlic and vegetables, adding the soy sauce.

Add the salmon and gently sauté in the liquid.

Cook and drain the noodles.

Serve the salmon on a bed of noodles with more chopped spring onions and sprinkle with the sesame seeds.

PASTA AND CHICKEN WITH ROCKET SALAD

This pesto chicken recipe is a perfect supper and can be varied by using either red or green pesto for two distinct tastes.

SERVES 2
PREPARATION TIME 5 mins
COOKING TIME 30 mins

2 organic chicken breast fillets
5 oz/125 g pasta – wholewheat, spelt or gluten-free,
   depending on taste
½ jar green or red pesto
rocket leaves

Cook the chicken breasts in the oven, about 15–20 minutes; when cooked, cool and cut into strips.

Meanwhile cook the pasta; allow to cool slightly, then add the chicken and pesto and mix. Reheat gently if necessary.

Serve and sprinkle with rocket leaves and add a generous pile as a side salad.

SPAGHETTI AND SAUCE WITH PARMESAN CHEESE

SERVES 2
SREPARATION TIME 5 mins
COOKING TIME 45–60 mins

5 oz/125 g spaghetti – wholewheat, spelt or gluten-free
3 tbsp extra virgin olive oil
1 large onion – chopped
2 garlic cloves – crushed
1 x 400 g can of chopped tomatoes
1 large handful basil leaves – shredded into small pieces
freshly ground black pepper
Parmesan or other hard cheese

Heat the oil in a pan and gently cook the onion and garlic.

Stir in the tomatoes and bring to a slow simmer; cook for 45–60 minutes. Add the basil and season.

Cook the pasta for 10 minutes or until *al dente*.

Serve the pasta and sauce with a generous sprinkle of Parmesan.

SNACKS

SUGAR-FREE WHOLEWHEAT MUFFINS

These are great if you want a healthy snack – you can add whatever you like in the form of dried or frozen fruit for a variety of flavours.

5 oz/125 g butter
1–2 tbsp stevia-based sweetener
2 medium eggs
5 oz/125 g plain wholemeal flour
1 tsp baking powder
1 tsp vanilla essence (optional)
approx 5 oz/125 g of any of the following – fresh or
    frozen strawberries, raspberries, blueberries;
    chopped dates, raisins; or 72% dark chocolate chips

Preheat the oven to 200 °C/400 °F/gas mark 6.

Cream the butter and sweetener in a large bowl.

Beat the eggs separately and mix with the butter.

Sieve the flour and baking powder and fold in. Stir in the vanilla essence.

Add your choice of fruit and mix gently.

Spoon the mixture into muffin cases and bake for about 18–20 minutes until risen and elastic to the touch.

SPELT AND HONEY COOKIES

A delicious yet nutritious treat.

PREPARATION TIME 5–10 mins
COOKING TIME 10–12 mins

  8 oz/200 g gwholegrain spelt flour
  1 tsp baking powder
  1 tsp ground cinnamon
  4 oz/100 g honey
  4 oz/100 g vegetable oil

Preheat oven to 190 °C/375 °F/gas mark 5.

Mix together all ingredients in a bowl to form a soft dough.

Grease a baking tray and place teaspoonfuls of the mix at intervals – they do tend to expand.

Bake in a preheated oven for 10–12 minutes or until golden.

POWER PROTEIN BARS

These are really simple to make – and don't need baking. Carry them with you to give you a protein boost after exercise or just as a healthy snack.

    17 oz/425 g dry oats or sugar-free muesli
    4 scoops whey protein powder (vanilla or chocolate)
    4 oz/100 g sugar-free peanut butter
    ¼ pint/120 ml of water or milk

    Optional additions
    dried fruit (raisins, cranberries, banana)
    seeds (pumpkin, sunflower, sesame, linseed)
    raw dark (72%+) chocolate chips or shavings

Note: If you add extra fruit or seeds, you may need more liquid.

Mix all the ingredients together in a bowl and then spread the mixture approx ½" thick over a baking tray or tin lined with greaseproof paper.

Put in the fridge for an hour or two and then cut into bars.

APPENDIX THREE:

JOURNAL

....

....

....

,

....

....

....

....

....

....

....

....

....

....

....

....

....

....

....

....

....

....

....

....

....

....

....

....

....

APPENDIX FOUR:
SUPPLIERS

United Kingdom

Organic Herbs and Spices

Steenbergs Organic – committed to Fairtrade, supplying a huge range of high-quality organic spices and organic cooking ingredients

6 Hallikeld Close
Barker Business Park
Melmerby
Ripon
HG4 5GZ
www.steenbergs.co.uk
T: +44 (0)1765 640088
F: +44 (0)1765 640101
Email: enquiries@steenbergs.co.uk

Kefir

Nourish Kefir – suppliers of ready-made drinks and starter sachets

PO Box 2891
Coulsdon
CR5 3WQ
T: 07973 627116
http://www.nourishkefir.co.uk/

Supplements, etc

Solgar UK Ltd
Aldbury
Tring
Herts
HP23 5PT
T: +44 (0)1442 890355
www.solgar.co.uk

My Protein – suppliers of high-quality protein powder,
creatine and coconut oil
T: +44 (0)845 094 9889
www.myprotein.co.uk

Sweeteners

Stevia-based sweetener – www.truvia.co.uk
or major supermarkets

United States

Organic Herbs and Spices

Oregon Spice Company – established in 1980, Oregon
Spice Company provides superior-quality herbs, spices and
custom blends.

13320 N.E. Jarrett Street
Portland, Oregon 97230
customerservice@oregonspice.com
Toll Free: (800) 565-1599
Local: (503) 238-0664
F: (503) 238-5585
http://www.oregonspice.com/

Kefir

Cultures for Health
13023 NE Highway 99 Suite 7–4
Vancouver WA 98686
T: 800-962-1959
http://www.culturesforhealth.com/

Supplements

Solgar, Inc.
500 Willow Tree Road
Leonia, NJ 07605
USA
T: 201-944-2311
F: 201-944-7351
Product information: 1-877-765-4274
www.solgar.com

Sweeteners

Stevia.com – online supplier of stevia-based products
http://www.stevia.com/

RECOMMENDED READING

Bass, Clarence, *Ripped*, Clarence Bass Ripped Enterprises, New Mexico, 1980

Bass, Clarence, *Lean for Life*, Clarence Bass Ripped Enterprises, New Mexico, 1992

Faulks, Martin, *Secrets of Rejuvenation*, Watkins Publishing, London, 2009

Faulks, Martin, *Butterfly Tai Chi*, Watkins Publishing, London, 2009

Faulks, Philippa, *Secrets of Meditation*, Watkins Publishing, London, 2009

Williams, Prof Mark & Penman, Dr Danny, *Mindfulness: A practical guide to finding peace in a frantic world*, Piatkus, London, 2011

http://www.crossfit.com/ Forging Elite Fitness. CrossFit is a core strength and conditioning programme.

http://zenhabits.net Zen Habits blog by Leo Babauta

INDEX